CORNER

OF THE

MIND

By

Roger R. Sigmon

Copyright 2017 Roger R. Sigmon

All rights reserved.

No part of this book may be reproduced, stored in a retrieval system, or transmitted by any means without the written permission of the author.

Cover Art is from public domain.

Cover idea and design created

by Roger R Sigmon

The views expressed in this work are solely those of the author and not necessarily those of the publisher, and the publisher hereby disclaims any responsibility for them.

Dedication

 I wish to dedicate this project to the memory of Ollie Sigmon. I realize this book does not begin to come close to capturing the amazing life this incredible lady lived. Hopefully it will continue her legacy. Also, to the memory of my father, Bobby Sigmon. He too departed much too soon. I dedicate this also to my family: Bobbie, Steve, Michelle, Chris, Janet, Barry, Christy, Jake, Lucas, and Liam. I trust this will be shared with future generations to preserve part of our family history.

 To my loving beautiful wife, Carol Sigmon and my wonderful stepdaughter Gracie. I pray we have many years together to grow as a family.

Table of Contents

Acknowledgements

There are so many friends, family, and others to thank for walking through this with me. First and foremost, I wish to thank God for allowing me to experience these events. I am thankful for the life I have been given and all the opportunities presented to me.

Carol Sigmon – for your support and encouragement, along with allowing me time to tackle this project. Pamela Mendoza Vallejo – for the encouragement and work you provided at the very beginning of the original project when it was just a jumbled mess of random thoughts. Melissa Haas – not only for years of friendship, but also for interest and encouragement throughout this long process. Aaron Bryant and Lee Swartz – for showing me how to make sense out of this crazy journey called life. Crystal Nadeau – for your friendship, chats, and phone calls as you helped me adjust to a new life in Tennessee. Stephany Hicks, Janie Hicks, Jeff Morrison, and Jennifer Morrison – for being there as we walked through some of the darkest moments of my life. Scott Harris, Kim Cox, and Steve Gregory – for teaching me about ministry through missions. David and Beverly Knox – for building a strong foundation of faith.

There are so many people to thank and acknowledge, yet space is limited. Please understand that I am thankful for all of you who are reading the words I have placed on paper. I would appreciate all feedback concerning what you read in this book. I would especially cherish stories of how this might have impacted you in anyway.

 It is my joy to see a dream come true. The writing of a book is quite an undertaking and is difficult work. I'm glad to have had so much encouragement and help along the way. I truly hope the efforts will pay off, and that the words contained within this book will be an encouragement to others. Once again, I say *thank you*!

Introduction

~

THE DAY TIME STOPPED

"He's not here right now; I'll tell him you called." Those words are forever burned into my memory as I suddenly realized life as I knew it would never be the same. I had been the caregiver for my mother, who was suffering from dementia, for just over a year. I had the opportunity to take some time off and to spend that time with my friend April in Panama City, Florida. Returning from the trip I had stopped at a highway rest stop in Columbia, South Carolina to call home to let Mom know I was only a few hours away and would be home soon.

I told her it was Roger, and I would be home in just a few hours – her response floored me. She told me to hold on and she would see if "Roger" was there. I was thinking *what? Huh?* She returned to the phone to tell me he was not there right now, but she would let him know I had called. I quietly said, *"Momma, it' me"* as the reality of her condition began to sink in.

No longer was the occasional memory lapse or hallucination the worst part. Now I was faced with the fact that she no longer recognized my name or voice. I walked back to my car in a total haze. I have no recollection of the remainder of the drive home. I could not shake off the cold chill that had suddenly overtaken every part of my body.

That phone call on a beautiful autumn day in 1998 would forever change my life.

The following is a collection of true events that transpired throughout a very difficult and dark period in my life. If you have ever known anyone who has suffered from Alzheimer's, then you will be able to relate to many of these stories. If you have ever lost anyone you love to death, then you will relate as well.

I have also included some very amazing experiences that I honestly feel can only be classified as miracles. I relay these and the other events in this book as a way of offering hope to anyone who might be experiencing the journey of a loved one with a terminal illness.

My goal is to let you know that you are not alone: others have gone and are going through similar pain. This is in no way meant to be a step-by-step process for grieving or to give quick and easy answers to dealing with loss. I am merely sharing the story of a remarkable lady and offering insights that I gleaned from having experienced these events.

Why the update you might ask. I felt there was more that needed to be said. I have watched several close friends experience the tragedy of losing loved ones. A few have had remarkable courage as they faced the inevitable. Most were lives cut much too short. I have always felt this book came close to being able to comfort and to heal, yet not close enough. I made the decision to undertake this rewriting to bridge that gap.

I originally wrote "Sleeping with the Angels" then closed the door to that era. I've only decided to reopen this door once more because there are things to be said that will help others. I don't talk much about this time in my life, for many years I have felt I said all I wanted and needed to say about it in the original book, however with the passage of time I realized more needed to be shared. I opened these old wounds, and released these ghosts of the memories once more in order that others may benefit and be comforted. Walking back through this door and embracing the pain of these memories at first is like pouring a container of salt into an open cut. Slowly it dawns on me it is more like hydrogen peroxide and the sting is necessary to remove the toxic infection and begin the healing.

Several life events have occurred during the almost seven years since the original release of this title. One of the biggest is now having a wife and stepdaughter. This new family has helped me to realize why we make the loving sacrifices that we do. It also reminds me that love can be painful as well. More importantly I am now able to see life through the lens of a parent. This minor adjustment in the pair of eyes I now utilize helps to focus on the drive behind a parent's unconditional love. In the end, you give all you can and trust you were able to pass along enough of the good to make a difference.

If you learn from anything in these chapters or know of someone who might, then please let them know about this book.

The North Carolina sun was scorching on that August afternoon as Ollie dipped her cotton-covered hands into a busted watermelon to clean them. Picking cotton was not a fun chore in the least. Each ball picked would leave behind a black sticky residue. Hands of the picker quickly became black and sticky. Watermelon juice was a quick in-the-field solution to removing the grime from hands. As the juice was flowing through her fingers, she daydreamed of leaving the life of the farm for adventure in the city. Maybe one day that tall, dashing, handsome, young man would come carry her away. Reality set in quickly as she and her sister Louise heard their father Jim, approaching. They knew it would mean trouble in all caps if he discovered they had destroyed one of Cleveland County's best watermelons just to rinse off their hands. He knew exactly how many were there and could tell from a mile away if one was missing.

The girls quickly gathered up their things and ran toward the house to see their mother. The aroma of Ada Belle's cooking was already filling the air. The wind carried the smell of homemade biscuits – the kind you can only find now in memories. No doubt there would be fresh fried chicken for dinner – "fresh" meaning that earlier that morning, Ada would have selected a hen from the yard and deemed it worthy of an honored spot on the table. In those days, a family didn't go to the corner grocery store meat department and buy a packaged chicken; it was all left up to the cook. This included catching the bird, wringing the neck, cleaning, and preparing.

This was life on the Porter farm in the 1930's and 1940's. Ollie was the next-to-youngest in a line of ten children. Life mostly consisted of rising before sunup to begin work in the fields, attend school, doing chores, and then going to bed. No iPhones, computers, nor television. It was not a bad life; the hard work instilled discipline, pride, and a good work ethic. The best escape was daydreaming.

Ollie's brother Charles has a different idea of escape. Whenever he would get into trouble he would run and hide under the house. There was enough room for him to fit, yet not enough for an adult. This worked only for so long, eventually he would get hungry or tired and still face his punishment anyway.

Many times, when she was around 13 or 14 years old, Ollie could be found standing beside the road waving as cars passed, dreaming that the dashing, young man from the city would sweep her away. She would usually wear a freshly picked flower behind her ear with her hair pulled back on one side. One must look her best when flirting with passing cars. Escapes such as these were few and far between though. One Fall she did find the time to play basketball at Falston School. I chuckle at this imagine knowing that as a full-grown adult she only stood 4' 11".

Jim and Ada Belle Porter were sharecroppers who raised cotton and watermelons in rural Cleveland County, North Carolina. He was also well known for making some of the best molasses in the state. No matter how tough times were or how little they had, a visitor would never leave from the Porter's empty-handed. Visitors and family were treated the same: you were always welcome. Jim and Ada Belle were two of the most generous people to ever live on the face of this earth. Unfortunately, today it is becoming rare to find people with the type of compassion these two simple, poor farmers possessed.

Jim (or JT as many knew him) might have looked a little scruffy on the outside, however his heart was pure gold. Most days he would forego shaving or even combing his hair. There was work needing to be done and no time to waste on those things. He was there to work the fields, not to impress anyone with his appearance. After all, would the blackbirds or field mice care if he had a three-day beard? As a kid, I can remember that he was always working whenever we would visit. Sometimes he would take a break from his work long enough to get a drink of water and say hello. That imagine would be the spark that ignited my own work ethic that at times borders on workaholic.

Hard work and hard times were no strangers. The Porters were no nonsense when it came to work. There was a time to work, and if the sun was up and there was no rain, the fields were the place to be. They knew the family depended on what that season's harvest would yield.

By the late 1940's, Ollie had met and fallen in love with the man of her dreams, Bobby R. Sigmon. The young man was tall and handsome. A hard worker with wavy, jet-black hair. He had no money, yet he was everything she had dreamed about. She eventually dropped out of high school in the 11th grade, and the two began a life together on December 9, 1950.

This was not the beginning of a fairy tale: this is the real world, and life is not always fair. Between the two of them, they had a grand total of $2. Their honeymoon was spent playing cards at the home of a couple who were friends of theirs.

Two years later after two previous miscarriages they gave birth to their first son, Steve, on December 19. This would not be the only change in their young marriage. Uncle Sam decided Bob was needed in the Korean War, so he watched the first few months of Steve's life through pictures. He was 8,800 miles from home, and Ollie was left alone to raise their son. Fortunately, by the mid 1950's the war was over, and the couple was reunited the following year after the United States withdrew from the country. He was discharged from the Army a few months later. The war had taken a toll on Bob's demeanor. He was a little more withdrawn and not as openly affectionate as before. He had seen many unspeakable things that would haunt him in nightmares for the rest of his life. Even so, the couple still loved until "death do us part".

Two more children, both were girls were born to Bob and Ollie. Things were now going much better, as there was now more income available from a new job for the growing family. However, as I stated, this is real life, and things are not always going to go well. By early 1962, Steve had developed a severe case of the flu. Eventually, this would develop into pneumonia, and eight-year-old Steve would breathe his last in February of that year.

The death of a firstborn child can be devastating. I could not even imagine how cheated Bob must have felt. He not only missed the first early years, but then his son was taken away much too soon. And Ollie... what mother can lose a child and not be forever changed? The remaining children, Bobbie, and Janet would have to learn at a very young age what death meant. No one will ever know what this loss truly meant for the four of them.

Friends and family talked Ollie into returning to work. There were still days when even the routine of work could not hide or ease the pain of a lost child. Some pain just never goes away. But regardless of this, she was a tough little lady and managed to keep going.

In early 1965, Bob and Ollie got some unexpected news: a baby was on the way! I'm sure there were some moments of questioning at first. The months to follow would be tense. How could the family survive if something happened to this child? The entire family was hoping and praying for a baby boy. They were not looking to replace Steve, yet they wished for the void of a brother and son to be filled. Then at a little past 5p.m. on Thursday, October 7, 1965, their newest son, Roger entered the world. God had granted their prayers for another male in the family, and this event would prove to be a great healing for Ollie. As, you can already gather, I am Roger.

Yes, it would have been very easy to become an incredibly spoiled, selfish, self-centered brat. Thankfully, the Lord gave me two sisters who didn't allow that to happen. My parents, siblings, and others did a good job of raising me so that I avoided those things. It was sometimes quite difficult trying to live up to unspoken expectations of "being Steve" or "being what Steve would have been." The Lord helped me very early on to understand that I was Roger and not Steve. I knew Steve had his purpose and I had mine.

I also understood the pain and heartbreak my parents had already endured. I always tried to live my life so that I would not cause them more hurt or shame. I was not the perfect child; however, I did my best to honor them. A special bond developed between me and the family. I always felt from a very young age that my purpose in life was to take care of my mother. She considered me a blessing from God; she had a chance to have her son back. This turn of events, as you can imagine, caused some jealousy in the family, but it was not serious. Everyone understood deep down why Ollie felt this way. I could not even imagine losing a child I loved dearly, and then unexpectedly be given another in his place. I believe I, too, would cherish every second of that precious gift.

Just to be clear, Ollie loved all her children and would have done anything to protect them. She may have only stood four-foot eleven, but if you ever crossed one of her children, you would have a fight on your hands. Family meant something to this lady, and she did her best to protect them.

The 1970's would bring about more trials and death. Between August 1973 and February 1974, the sting of death would strike not once, not twice, but three times. Bob's father, Ray would die; followed by Ollie's mother, Ada Belle; and finally, her father, Jim. In just the short span of eleven years, Ollie had lost her firstborn son, her father-in-law, and both parents.

Many times, I would see her as she laid across the bed, her eyes red from crying. I knew of nothing to do but to put my arms around her and give her a hug. I could not understand completely how she felt, yet I knew she was hurting and needed love. The passage of time helps to heal these types of wounds. Things would eventually get back to an appearance of normal.

Tragedy would once again strike in the 1990's. Bob became rather ill with a severe cold and upper back pain in the fall of 1994. He went to numerous doctors and had countless tests run. He felt lifeless, depressed, uninterested in most anything, and had almost no appetite. A doctor had a hunch about what the problem might be and sent him to a specialist. The hunch was correct. After three days in the hospital in May 1995, the diagnosis came back. He was suffering from what was then a very rare form of lung cancer called mesothelioma. Unfortunately, it was untreatable and had no known cure. The worst news was that Bob only had four to six weeks to live at this point, which meant he might not live pass the week of July 4.

Ollie had always been a strong survivor and she became the sweetest nurse to her husband. I never saw two people grow so close in such a short time. It was so obvious that no matter what differences they had faced, they were now going to enjoy the rest of the time they had together.

Bob was a great patient and a fighter. He fought hard to hang on and endured extreme pain in order not to worry his wife or family. He never gave up, and he even had a game plan to getting better. By this time, I was even convinced that maybe God was going to heal him to show His power. I had told Ollie that it would be so incredible to share such a story of healing. However, it was not to be. Friday, June 9, 1995, the entire family was gathered at Mom and Dad's house. It was obvious he knew his time was very near, as he began to go around the room, giving each of us what would be, in essence his last words. I don't think anyone ate very much of the pizza we had ordered, no one seemed very hungry.

I vividly remember watching him stare blankly at the Braves game on television, trying to comprehend what was going on in the game. Bob was a huge baseball fan and loved the Braves, Red Sox, and American Legion Post 100 baseball. The braves would go onto win the World Series that fall.

Many times, we hear people compare our relationship to God as that of a father to a son or daughter. The question that will eventually arise is, what if that father-child relationship is strained or nonexistent? This can be a difficult role for some to understand if they have never experienced that type of role on earth. Hopefully at least one parent has set a good example of parental love to show their children how this order of love should be. I was fortunate enough to have had two parents who demonstrated this kind of love. They both had very different ways of showing this love, yet I knew it was there and recognized it.

There were times when my relationship with my father was not the best, and several times I questioned his love for me or mine for him. This mainly came from both of us being male and from having a simple misunderstanding or personalities. Fortunately, we worked out any differences we had and thus enjoyed a good father-son relationship.

Tragedy and pain were the two things that really sealed our relationship. In 1994 when my wife left me, my dad was also crushed by the news. I was surprised at just how hard the news hit him. I realized he was hurting for me. His love was deep enough and strong enough for me that, as I went through a very difficult time, he had the ability to share it with me.

We had gained a respect and love for one another by this time, and it meant so much to me for my dad to walk through this with me. We had always watched sports together, mostly on television. I was always the diehard optimist thinking that if there was time left on the clock, there was still time to pull out a come-from behind victory. It was not always the outcome, yet I never gave up hope. I remember one Fall we were watching a Redskins game. Mathematically they had a chance to pull out the game, yet it would take a tremendous amount of good fortune to pull it off.

I kept saying as they inched back into the game that they were going to be able to do it. My dad just said, "I would like to see that too, but they don't have enough time." I kept on with my opinion that they barely had enough time left, yet it was still enough if this or that happened in this amount of time etc. Long story short: they pulled out the victory, and of course, I was thrilled they won, and I had been right. Instead of my dad getting mad at being wrong, he just humbly said, "guess they had enough time after all." This type of scenario would play more into our relationship than I could ever dream possible. As he was dying, he never once began to give up. He had learned to fight against hopeless odds by watching my behavior even through something as meaningless as sports. The lesson was not lost on him. It was still tough to watch him suffer through pain so intense that even after the legal dose of morphine, he still in pain and had a need for more medication. He never knew how serious his condition was until hospice arrived to deliver a hospital bed. Dad had spent enough time at the bedside of cancer patients to know this was normally a sign that the patient would be made comfortable as they prepared to transition from one life to the next. It would only initially faze him then he resolved to fight even harder. He was determined to win!

Now I could be there for him, so I could share his pain as he had shared mine earlier. It's a helpless feeling when there seems to be nothing you can do. One Sunday afternoon, he asked me to pray for him. I was not sure if he meant to pray *with* him or *for* him, so I asked just to be sure. He wanted me to pray for him. I was touched beyond words just by the thought that he put enough respect and trust into my prayers and relationship with God that he wanted me to pray on his behalf. I remembered that only a year or two earlier, he had prayed over me as I was ordained as a deacon, and now I was praying over him as he was preparing to let go of this life. I could not for a million dollars tell you one word I prayed other than maybe "Dear Lord" and "Amen" anything else I do not recall. I just prayed from my heart, and I admit I never felt closer to God or my dad than I did at that moment. After we prayed, he asked me to rub lotion onto his back. I had to be careful, because although the lotion was soothing, too much pressure caused pain. As I applied the lotion, my thoughts were not really in that moment. I knew it would probably be the last time I did this for him; however, I never realized this would be the very last time we would be together with him awake. Soon after this, I left Dad to attend the evening church service. This was June 11, 1995.

  Normally I would have eaten dinner after church with a group of friends, but instead, I went to visit my parents. Dad was asleep when I got there, and I did not wish to wake him, so I kissed his cheek and told him I loved him. I found out that several of my friends had stopped by to see Dad before church, and he had asked them if they had seen "his boy." At the time, everyone just assumed he was asking to see me. This could have very well been the case. Keep in mind his first-born son had died over thirty years before this. I must wonder if possibly he knew he was about to leave this world and enter the next soon. Could he have been already preparing to meet his son that he had been separated from for over three decades?

My wife Carol, and I have discussed many times if people near either get a visit from a departed loved one or if they are granted a glimpse behind the veil that separates this world from the next. She has had family members claim to have talked with or seen other family just prior to their own deaths. I remember when my grandfather (my dad's father) was dying, he claimed to have seen and talked with his brother Eugene and my brother Steve. He said they had set on the edge of the bed and talked with him. Everyone assumed that he had seen his reflection in the mirror and thought that was his brother, they looked very much alike and that he thought I was Steve since we also looked very much alike. They told him this and adamant that it happened, and it was who he said they were. He died a few days later and that has stuck in my mind for forty plus years. Why do we hear so many stories like this? How could it even be possible? So, is it possible different realms or dimensions overlap or merge?   I'm just bringing this up as an interesting question and to prove we really have limited information on what a dying person truly experiences. You can make your own conclusions about this matter.

Shortly after 6:00a.m. on Monday, June 12, Bob lost his battle. Although this was a terrible loss for our family, we knew he would enter heaven. This truth seemed to bring peace to Ollie. Although obviously upset and grieving, I never noticed her losing hope. I truly believe knowing he was eternally safe was enough to keep her hanging on.

Through all these tragedies, Ollie was always a woman of great faith. She knew God was in charge, and He could make anything at all happen. She also knew God didn't always answer our prayers in the way we wanted. She was okay with that. Many times, I heard her speak of how God had His angels placed around us to protect us. There is no doubt she had a very strong faith in God and angels. He was very real to her, and she wanted Him to real to others as well.

She lived through many trying times. There is not a time I can ever recall her feeling sorry for herself. She had the ability to roll with whatever life threw her way. I'm sure inside she felt like dying many times, yet one would never know it by being around her. Ollie was always upbeat no matter what the circumstance.

Ollie loved her family very much. She was always around to lend her support. This little lady was a very proud mother, and she took great pride in the accomplishments of each of her children. She was by far their biggest cheerleader. I have never known anyone who could find an encouraging word in any circumstance the way she could.

It seemed that almost everyone she met became her friend. It is rare to find someone that you instantly like, and fortunately, she happened to be one of those people. To my knowledge, she had no enemies only a large circle of friends. There are some people that you just feel better by being around, and this was Ollie. The one theme that runs through comments from people who knew her during various stages of her life is that she was a sweet, lovable person who was always there for her friends and family.

Chapter Two

JIM AND ADA PORTER

I briefly mentioned a few of the characteristics of my grandma and grandpa Porter in the previous chapter. I hope by sharing a few stories that it will paint a much clearer picture of the remarkable people I was able to share a few short years with.

I visited their former home a few years ago, and recently I shared a few stories of that home with my sisters. As we shared about the house and our grandparents, a story of their lives began to be woven through the tales. It seemed all our memories were fond ones. The main theme seemed to be that these were generous and loving people.

During that visit, I had shared with them my dream of one day restoring the house to its original design. That may or may not ever happen, yet it opened dialogue about the home and the people who once lived there. During that return visit to memories of old I could still hear and see the ghost of years long past on the wind. The landscape had changed, no longer did the fields burst forth with life sustaining produce. A few scraggly weeds were tossed about by the breeze, mocking the once lush fields. The house had seen it's better days as well. A few haphazard attempts at addon additions and renovation had altered the home of my childhood memories. I did spend a few minutes talking with the current residents. I told them about spending time there as a kid in the early 70's. They found that to be cool as I pointed out which fields yielded which crops. Some of the land had been redeveloped, thus erasing some of the fields and hidden areas we played in as kids. My new friends told me to take my time revisiting days gone by. I did just that and snapped a few photos as well.

My sisters and I talked about some of the things we remembered about the house as kids. Central air and heat were not very common in that area in the early 1970s. The house was heated by a wood-burning stove in the front room. This room served as both a living room and bedroom during the cold winter months. Even though there was no air conditioning, I never remember feeling hot when I visited.

The most common form of air conditioning was window units. I miss the days before people became so spoiled with air conditioning. It seems now if the room temperature is not set below sixty degrees, people whine about it being too hot.

My grandparents leased the home and land they lived on. Most of that payment was made by sharecropping and money made from what the fields yielded. I'm sure they were taken advantage of through this arrangement; however, they were very poor, trusting people. As a child, this property was ideal for spending hours exploring. There were woods, dirt roads, creeks, barns, stables of some sort, and endless fields of farmland. And stray cats were everywhere. I'm sure they all ventured to that area because of the fact where there are crops and fields, there are mice.

The property was also home to beautiful domestic flowers, wildflowers, and trees and some very green grass. This was the country, and it was so removed and peaceful. The view from the house across the fields was also marvelous.

The memories transport me to a more ideal time. This was an era when a man's word meant something. A person said they would do something, and it meant they would do it, not just consider it. People were more generous and honest. There was crime and dishonesty also, yet these types were not as widespread as today. People didn't even lock their doors or windows. I cannot even begin to imagine leaving a window or door unlock today.

My grandparents were very generous people who would always share what they had with others. They were dirt-poor farmers who truly made their living off the land, yet you would have thought they were the richest people on earth by how much they would give away. I never recall a time we left without a jar of molasses, watermelon, cantaloupe, green beans, or whatever they had to share. One never left their house empty-handed.

I remember very well three items my grandfather gave to me. He had a trunk that sat under a window in the living room. Twice he went into that trunk and gave me an item each time. The first was a pocket watch with a leather strap that I carried with me to school for several years.

Everyone else had wristwatches, yet I had my special pocket watch. One other kid really thought my watch was cool, and he showed up with one a few days later. Another item from the trunk was obviously from the flea market a few miles from their home. It was a toy outhouse with a little boy peeing inside. A small bubble on the outside was pressed and he would spray water. I thought this was hilarious, but I don't think my parents were as amused as I was by this new toy.

The living room had a black-and-white TV that sat to the right of the trunk. I remember going there on Sunday afternoons, and I would watch Fred Kirby as he introduced episodes of *the Little Rascals*. Fred Kirby was my hero, the only cowboy I liked. I always pulled for the Indians in any cowboy movie; however, Fred was a cowboy I could like. We had a color TV at home, so I knew he wore a red cowboy shirt with white fringe. One Saturday we were visiting my grandparents, and my grandfather wanted my mother to drive him to Shelby. He insisted I go with them. I remember parking on the street and him going into a store and coming back out with a box.

The box held the sacred Fred Kirby cowboy suit complete with shirt, pants, and hat. The best part was that it was for *me*! I have no idea how much that cost him and why he felt the need to buy such an expensive gift for me, yet forty years later, I can recall it as if it were this past Saturday. I can only imagine that he bought this for me after seeing how fascinated I was with watching *the Little Rascals* and Fred Kirby each week. In any case, it was a truly unexpected and very much appreciated gift. I wore that treasured shirt to school one time, but the fringe and a room full of first graders was not a good combination. Some of the fringe did not make it through the day. It was just too much of a temptation for some of the kids to leave alone. I still feel the sadness from realizing the fringe could never be reattached to the shirt, even though I had saved as many as I could to take home to my mom. I am puzzled to this day as to why the teacher did not put a stop to the fringe pulling.

A memory my sister shared with me is that after my brother died, my family lived with my grandparents for a short time. I was not yet born, so I have no idea of what life was like there. I would have loved the opportunity to have stayed with them for an extended time. She shared with me that our family took a TV over there and that they would watch a movie sometimes at night. I believe movies were only shown a few nights a week on the three networks. (Yes, there was a time when only three channels were on a TV.) My grandparents basically woke up and went to bed with the sun. Being farmers, their days and lives were centered around daylight.

My grandmother would begin watching the movie with them, yet seldom got to see the end of it. Grandpa would enter the room wearing his nightshirt and announcing, "Ada [he pronounced it Ader], it's time for bed." After a few replays of this, she would give in and go to bed. I believe her attraction to seeing a movie might have been due to the fact she was an avid reader. this allowed her to see a story played out in real time, not just unfolded in her mind.

I heard stories of my sisters watching my grandfather make molasses during their stay. He had two mules that would pull a contraption that operated part of the machinery in the process. I know he grew his own sugar cane, and basically everything that went into the molasses was grown on their farm. I would so love to have witnessed this process. So many things from a generation or two ago have been lost. Almost everything today is imported or mass-produced. There was an art to making things such as molasses. Simple skills are passed down from generation to generation, yet it only takes one generation to stop making something and hundreds of years of skill and tradition are lost. People of my grandparents' generation were survivors. Makes me wonder if something happened to our technology and we were thrown back into a survival mode, if there would be enough people around with the knowledge and skill to keep life going.

My grandfather loved to drink, and I would dare say there was probably a moonshine still or two on the property. I recall once riding in the car as my parents took my grandfather to a place called The Red Door to buy a beer. Yes, there was a time when grocery stores and convenience stores could not sell alcohol. I was not allowed to go in with my grandfather, so I sat in the backseat awaiting his return. He came back out with a brown paper bag containing a Pabst Blue Ribbon beer. I was too young to know what beer was exactly. The thing I remember the most is my dad telling Grandpa in a stern voice, "Jim, do not open that in the car, it would get me in serious trouble."

I was rather confused as to why my grandfather would buy something that might get my father in trouble. Knowing that he had something that was bad for so many people, I believe helped form my distain for alcohol from a very early age. I was probably three or four years old during this time. Alcohol has never had any appeal to me, and I can count on one hand the number of times I have ever even tasted any form of alcohol.

Several years later Jim Porter would walk down the aisle of a church and then walk away from a habit that owned his life for many years. I don't know if he was abusive or mean when he was drunk; I have never really heard any of those stories. I do know that his family worried about what might happen to him when he went to Shelby to get drunk. He was well known as a successful producer of cotton, watermelons, molasses, corn, and strawberries. This meant he would go to town to sell his wares, and many taxi drivers and others would be aware he had all his earnings with him.

The only fl aw I ever have heard about this man was his battle with alcohol. I did not quite understand what it meant when, as a small child, I heard he had been saved from alcohol. I only knew it had something to do with Jesus and no more drinking. The saddest part of his addiction to alcohol was that some of his hard-earned money was easily parted from him, and there was less to give back to his family. But then he somehow overcame this when the story of Christ's love got through to him. I'm not sure if it was someone's life, he had been influenced by or maybe even a sermon he had heard; I only know he was pursued by God and eventually stopped running from Him. I wish it were possible to sit down with him and hear his story; it would be so amazing to hear this from him.

I do not remember for sure if this was before or after my grandmother's onset of Alzheimer's and eventual placement in a nursing home. I remember always seeing her doing one of three things: either she was cooking, working in the yard, or reading her Bible. I know the Bible was something she loved to read. In fact, she loved reading just about anything. She read newspapers, the Bible, comic books I would bring to her house, and even the box of a train puzzle I had taken over there to work on. I guess there is no reason to wonder where my love of reading came from.

I have searched my memory, and never once did I hear my grandparents ever lament about being poor. I'm not even sure if they knew they were poor. They knew their role in life and lived it well. I keep saying they were simple people, and they were. They always seemed to be content. their work ethic seems to be the one thing that stands out in my mind. They were hard workers, yet it was not to accumulate things; it was to survive. They lived harvest to harvest, and if the fields did not produce, they might starve. They wore work clothes and had no car. They had very little furniture and a hand-me-down black-and-white TV, yet they were completely satisfied with this lifestyle. When I recall the Porters, I will always remember they were not afraid to work and were generous beyond belief.

There is an old saying to never forget where you came from. I can say that by revisiting the past of your family, it may help you understand more about the way you are wired. My parents and both sets of grandparents were hard workers, and I guess that is why I have very little patience with people who don't work hard or who just want to show up and collect a paycheck.

 I'm not bragging, only stating that this is part of my heritage, and I do take lessons from the past. I'm proud to say that I have the same blood flowing through my veins of such wonderful people who helped make this country great. People like Jim and Ada Porter helped set the standard in this nation, and we could use more like them today. I like their version of the American Dream much better than the version that is being presented and pursued today.

Chapter Three

~

OLLIE

A chapter devoted to the person that an entire book centers around must seem rather odd. I wanted to take just a moment to help you understand a little more of the lady behind the story. I've included many things about her life in the other chapters yet wanted to say more about her interaction with her family and friends.

Ollie truly enjoyed traveling, she loved country and gospel music. Naturally, her favorite destination was Nashville, TN. Surprising one of her father places there was Printer's Alley. She didn't care for the risqué cafés or the dive bars, however she couldn't get enough of live music. Printer's Alley has sadly fallen victim to the same "progress" in Nashville that has either destroyed or greatly reimaged much of Music Row and other historic areas of a city that can trace its' roots back to music, namely country music.

My parents had discovered a venue in Kings Mountain, NC called Crossroads Music Park. There each weekend live country music could be found and several times per month well known county music stars such as George Jones, Conway Twitty, Loretta Lynn, Dolly Parton, Porter Wagoner, and many others would appear. The main emcee of this venue which was owned by Tom Brooks was Willard Boyles. He along with his wife Melba soon formed a tour business that they named Willard's Tours and Nashville was a common destination. My parents began traveling with this tour group and fell in love with Nashville. Willard worked as a disc jockey at WKMT 1220 AM, which was a country station at that time. One of his fellow dee jays was Jim Arp, that became a family friend as well. Jim performed several times at Crossroads, released a few singles, and had at one point been in the band for Seals and Croft. I had a passion and love for radio and a dream of being a dee jay and my mom also shared that same dream for herself. Jim was kind enough to teach her how to run the board and let her do a brief amount of reading news and introducing a few records.

Another passion she had that she later abandoned later in life, but passed onto me and two of her grandchildren was writing. Her draw was to poems and songs. As a teenager, she wrote many poems and songs, she even entered a song into a contest at the Cleveland County Fair. She never heard anything from the judges, however she later heard a song on the radio which she said soundly strikingly familiar to hers. Who knows, maybe it was or maybe not.

My dad worked on various shifts, rarely first shift, so she and I had to entertain ourselves during the evening hours. One of the things we did was write songs, or at least we called them songs. I would love to have those precious words now, unfortunately they are all lost forever. What I do have is a passion and talent for writing thanks to her example and participation. That led to me writing short stories, and later books. She gave me the nudge to explore writing and to never sell myself short for that I am forever grateful. I have a niece and a nephew that both dabbled in creative writing, both have talent but have never pursued it as more than just a hobby.

The poems, songs, and short stories I wrote with my mother and on my own fell victim to improper storage and pests in the storage area of a former apartment I lived in. When I was a teenager, I remember my mom passing along a few of her songs to a local singer/songwriter that made frequent trips to Nashville. I realize she was trying to help him and not looking for a ticket to fame, however I knew she had made a mistake as I watched him take her work and fold it into his back pocket. I'm sure they never made it out of Crossroads Music Park that night unless it was in the trash. I have no clue if what she wrote was anything more than ramblings, yet it would have been nice if this budding country music artist had shown her work a little more respect. He died a few years later, so no idea whatever became of those lyrics.

I realized just how ingrained generosity was in my mom one Sunday afternoon when my friend Jamie had stopped by the house to work on a problem with the power. This was in the early stages of her dementia, yet she was beginning to get confused. She had always wanted to make sure people left with something, she asked Jamie if he wanted some white donuts and kept trying to hand him something in a paper towel. He looked at me quizzically and I told him go ahead and take them. She was handing him white Danish wedding cookies, that why "white donuts" was not connecting with him.

A few months later we I took Mom to the Hong Kong Lobsteer Inn, which was a Chinese Buffet. We both enjoyed Chinese food, so we took advantage of the inexpensive midday buffet. I noticed her cheeks began to enlarge and resembled a chipmunk, then it dawned on me she was not swallowing her food, even though she kept putting more in. I finally convinced her to swallow before eating anymore. It was somewhat comical, yet I began to wonder just what might be happening to cause this.

A mother always has a special bond with and love for her children that's what makes her a mom. Fathers might love their children just as much, but there are times when only a mom knows how to handle a situation; it's part of their role in the family. Men and women are very different, and both parents are needed for proper balance in raising a child. I was fortunate enough to have both parents in my home something many children today are not afforded due to various reasons.

Something about the presence of a mom makes a house a home. I can remember the difference when my mother would come home from work. My dad even watched the clock, waiting for her time to arrive. Ollie was just that type of person her presence made a difference. She walked into a room and the mood changed for the better. She was one of those people that other people loved to be around.

I feel this to be a result of the fact that she had absolutely no prejudice of any kind toward anyone. She saw people, not types of people or colors of people just people. It seems everyone has some form of prejudice in them at some level, yet I could never detect it in her.

The word *integrity* was defined through her life. She did not believe in lying; and as far as I know, she never told a lie purposely. Truth was important and truth was what was spoken. Ollie had a way of making everything sound positive. I'm sure this is where I learned the ability to always be positive and see the world from a glass-half-full perspective.

Ollie was a farm girl raised in the rural South with hardly any money as a child and not much more as an adult. She never complained about being poor; Ollie thought being poor was more a state of mind than a bank account balance. When it came to giving love and support, she was one of the richest people I have ever known. She may not have been able to help financially, but you could count on her praying for you and encouraging you.

Recently, a good friend from my young-adult days made a statement that really meant a lot to me. During my early college days, my then best friend Rodney Jeffries was playing shortstop for Bessemer City High School and Cherryville Post 100 American Legion baseball. We would go to support him, and my mom and her friend Jackie Willis became two of Rodney's biggest fans. That was in the late 1980s. In 2011, Rodney still remembered her support, and he told me how much that had meant to

him to have my mom at all his games. Rodney had stopped by the house one day on his way to or from somewhere and my mom asked him for his autograph. He laughed and smiled then said, "you're serious"? She said of course she was, and she wanted it because she believed in him and wasn't sure if she could get his autograph after he made it to the major leagues. Although Rodney had great talent and a few tryouts for the pros he never got the call. He did go onto become a successful body builder and personal fitness trainer.

It was also Rodney's mother, Ruby Jeffries, who would bring me to tears at my mother's graveside by letting me know how important it was to her that my mother was one of the first people to truly welcome her and make her feel at home at the church we were attending. The fact that it was a predominately white congregation and the Jeffries were African American made an impact on me through her statement. Being involved in athletics, it was normal for me to have a diverse group of friends. It never really occurred to me that I had teammates and friends who were African American, Asian, Hispanic, or Caucasian. They were just friends and teammates. Putting into perspective the generation that our parents had been raised in, I realized we were not that far removed from segregation. The open acknowledgment of my mother's nonbiased acceptance of people of any walk of life truly touched my heart. It had never been much clearer than in that moment. As I stood there sobbing and hugging Miss Ruby, she comforted me as a mother would have.

Ollie's love for us kids was always obvious, yet she still liked to do nice things for us. I will never forget how she would bring me a moon pie and Orange Crush home from work. Keep in mind that we didn't have much money, and she probably used her break money to get this for me. She knew it made me happy, and that made her happy. That is what true love is all about: doing something for someone just to make them happy no strings attached. Truly putting the other person's wants and needs before your own is what matters. Even the smallest or the simplest of acts can make a lifetime of difference. I still laugh every time I think of her saying,

"The good Lord will probably never give me any money because I would just give it away." She wasn't saying this to brag or draw attention to herself; she was just stating a fact. I am convinced had she ever won a million dollars, she would have given 10 percent to the church, split a portion three ways among her children, and given away the remainder to anyone who was in need. Money really meant nothing to her—not the way it does to some people anyway.

I have tried to learn from this example, and although I have not achieved Mom's standard yet, I do a decent job. I try to be a good steward of my money. I attempt to not spend money on myself or things that are not really that important needs more than wants. Sometimes the wants win out and I spend money on things I later realize was a waste. I prefer to use my money toward helping others and organizations that help others. I'm not as good at this as I would like to be, but I'm working on it. I had two tremendous role models in my parents who lived this out for me, so at least I have an idea of what it looks like.

I've heard many times that Christ followers should be showing others "Jesus with skin on." Well, this is something I saw that was being lived out each day of my mother's life. She always had a smile no matter how she felt, and she would always be there for family, friends, or strangers. I only heard encouraging words come from her mouth, never a negative comment or put-down to anyone. During her funeral, Rev. Andy Raines made the comment that he enjoyed watching Ollie worship. She knew she was in the house of the Lord to worship, yet she also knew that following Christ was a lifestyle and not just a Sunday morning or Wednesday night event. My mother was fully aware that the church was not a building; it was a group of believers doing life together, showing Christ to others.

  The older I get, the more I realize how blessed I am to have been placed in the family I was born into. I find it difficult to imagine having any better combination of parents than what I had. They were not perfect, yet they were perfect for me, faults, and all. Perfect parents would not have been able to shape me into the man I am becoming. I learned as much through their bad points as their good points.

  Having been blessed with a wonderful wife and stepdaughter, I hope to leave the same legacy with them my parents left for me. I would feel like a successful parent if my family could see that even though I was imperfect, I loved them with all my heart and did my very best to protect and teach them. I hope they will be able to say I lived out a Christ like action for them and that my lifestyle spoke more to them in a positive way than anything I could have ever tried to teach them through words.

We've all heard that actions speak louder than words. It is true. I remember someone saying when I was younger that their kids might not always hear what they are saying, but they will sure hear what they say through their actions. I must say I would agree with this statement.

My parents were consistent through their actions and lifestyles with what they told us. I can only imagine they were just modeling the same type of parenting that they received from their parents. I truly wish I could have paid closer attention to what they were saying and doing when I was much younger. I could have learned more from them than having to learn it on my own the hard way. There were many times I misunderstood actions of my father; however, as I become more and more like him each day, I truly understand.

If I can give any advice to children of any age, I would say at least hear your parents out. They have lived longer and experienced more than you. They love you very much, and all they are trying to do is help you avoid pain and mistakes. They have already been down that road and only want to warn you of which sinkholes to avoid.

As I write this, I can see God through my parents' lives. It's amazing how they can still teach me, even many years after their deaths. Many days I wish for nothing more than to just sit and talk with my parents to share with them what is going on in my life and how much I learned from them. Just to tell them I love them and hear them tell me they are proud of me. Fortunately, these were conversations that did take place while there was still time. Reliving it once more would be fantastic.

I'll just say: leave nothing unsaid, and if ever anything regrettable has been said, then by all means correct that situation before it is too late. Most of all, live each day of your life as if it is your last. Never do anything that you would be ashamed to have as anyone's last memory of you.

Chapter Four

~

THE ONSET: ROLE REVERSAL

May 1996, I put my home on the market at the request of my former wife. She intended to buy a new home with her current husband and needed to remove this mortgage from her credit record. I did not wish to move; however, this would turn out to be a huge blessing in disguise. The house was only on the market a few hours before the very first couple to view it decided to make an offer. After the closing, I moved in with my mother. She had never said anything before, yet I knew she did not like living alone after the death of my father the year before.

The following month, we used some of the escrow from the sale of the home to go to the Country Music Fan Fair in Nashville, Tennessee. The event was taking place during the one-year anniversary of my father's death, and I knew this would be an excellent way to keep my mother's mind occupied. This would also mark the first visit to Nashville she had taken since the death of my father. They always visited there each year at least twice. My parents loved music, and what more appropriate place to enjoy visiting than Music City, USA?

During the week, we had the opportunity to visit with some of the artists that we both enjoyed. She was really hoping that Garth Brooks would make a surprise appearance, even though he was not scheduled to be at the events during the week. I made sure to find out where any of her favorite artists were appearing, so she could have a chance to meet and chat with them.

We had made this trip with a tour group I found through an advertisement. Several of the people had been to Fan Fair in Nashville many times and offered tips to those making their first trip. It soon became apparent that some people still wanted to hold out on a few tips to allow themselves a better chance at meeting artists that were more difficult to see.

Unfortunately, we found out a few hours too late that Garth Brooks had indeed shown up unannounced the previous afternoon and had stayed for a record, thirty-six straight hours to make sure everyone in line got to meet him. A few ladies from our group had found out he was there and decided to keep the information to themselves instead of sharing with anyone else in the group. Even without meeting him, she was still able to have a very enjoyable trip, and we accomplished the main goal of not letting the anniversary of a death become a depressing negative time.

I began to take care of Mom's financial affairs. She had very few debts, however, she also had very little income. Each month I had to help her out financially so she could meet her obligations. I was also still in the process of paying off some debt incurred during my marriage. I was now responsible for paying the bills of three people.

The stress from this was building, yet I kept doing everything in my power to stay on top of our finances.

Mom kept forgetting to record debits or checks in the checkbook register, which made it more difficult to keep track of the cash flow. At that point, one of her brothers offered to help her out with some money. I had recently traded cars to reduce my monthly car payment and to release myself from a car loan that carried a co-signer, which was my ex-wife. My Uncle and his family, however, were convinced I had used my mother's money to purchase this car. It was just so amazing to me that people could come up with such ridiculous thoughts. I was spending every cent I could make to cover the debts of three people, and yet I was being accused of stealing money from someone who didn't even have money. I just let it go and continued living my life, letting them form whatever opinion they wished to form. I had too many other things keeping me occupied.

During the next year or so, we began noticing that Mom was becoming a little forgetful about a few things. No one really thought anything about this, thinking it was just a part of getting older. She was in her sixties, yet everyone knows that as we age the mind changes, so our family thought it was no big deal.

Soon she began to move beyond just forgetting simple things like where she had placed her keys. It seemed now that every few days she would be a little confused after waking in the morning or from a nap. It was a similar feeling to that sensation you have when you take a nap on an afternoon when you are really tired and wake disoriented as to what time or day it is. This would only last a few seconds, and it only happened a few times a week at most. Again, we really didn't think there was anything wrong. She was retired, so without a workweek routine, we could see how it would be easy to lose track of days.

I noticed she was writing more notes to help her remember certain things, and she would look at the newspaper each morning to see what date it was. In hindsight, all these things were warning signs; however, in real time it just does not add up as quickly.

Things began to change at a much more rapid pace. We visited my Uncle Dennis and Aunt Louise in May of 1997, and by now it was becoming more noticeable that she was easily confused. We had gone there to see a concert festival at North Carolina State University. During this visit, Mom had gotten up a few times during the night and then gone back to bed. When we got back home, she seemed to not know exactly that we were back. She didn't say that outright, yet some of her actions seemed to indicate this.

We returned to Nashville a few weeks later Fan Fair had now become a tradition for us over the last three years. I now knew a few artists who were just breaking into the business, and we were going to attend their fan club parties. During some of the meet-and-greet sessions at the fairgrounds, a few of the artists that we met seemed to notice things were not quite as they should be with her. I took her photo with Vern Gosdin, and she stood there a second as if she had no clue where she was or what she was doing. Later after we had talked with John Connelly, he pulled me to the side and said for me to "take care of Mom." I thought that sort of odd at the moment; then would later realize that from the outside it was much more obvious that she was no longer in a normal mental state.

In the hotel, a few nights I awoke to find my mother going through the drawers. I asked her what she was doing, and she said she was putting away the pots and pans. I assumed she was just sleepwalking, so I played along and guided her back to bed. The seriousness of the situation would first dawn on me near the end of the week. We were at the MCA show at the fairgrounds and Olivia Newton-John was the main artist. I told Mom to stay in the seat, and I would be back in about five minutes, I was going to walk through the photo line, and when I got back we could leave. She seemed very coherent and said that would be fine.

I quickly went through the line, and when I returned to our section, she was nowhere in sight. I'm sure I looked like a deer in headlights, as I quickly scanned the section, we had been sitting in. The gentleman seated behind us said she left toward the gate just before I got back. I don't normally panic; however, the thought struck me that twenty-five thousand people were there, and they would all be heading out the same exit in just a matter of minutes. I instinctively said a short prayer sort of along the lines of "*help*." Only through the grace of God did I spot her walking a few feet ahead of me and in the general direction of our car. I caught up to her just as the crowd was beginning to exit. When I asked why she had not waited, she said, "I thought you were waiting in the car." The next night we were going to Chely Wright's fan club party, and I made sure that I had someone to help me keep an eye on her. I didn't leave her side without asking someone to make sure she didn't wander off. Jennifer, a girl I had met through the fan club, was a godsend by taking the time to just chat with Mom for a few minutes to allow me to go grab us some food and have a little break.

This party was in a gym of a local Nashville school, so basketball was being played after Chely's concert. As members mingled and played basketball, Chely visited with a few people in the stands. I did not know that she had spent so much time with my mother until later when Mom told me about the conversation.

Driving back to our hotel, Mom kept talking about the girl who asked about her makeup and commented on her fingernail polish. She said that the same girl had asked about her experience with Fan Fair and her interest in music and countless other things. My mom talked about how long she had talked. I thought at first she had meant that it was Jennifer she had been talking to, but Mom then said it was later. This made no sense to me, because I knew I had not been gone long enough getting food for all that to have happened. I asked her what girl she was talking about, and she said, "When you played basketball, the girl we watched sing came over and sat down."

I had asked an older couple that was there to keep an eye on her while I participated in a quick free-throw shooting contest. I think I had the worst shooting game of my life. I was constantly looking back to see if she was all right concentrating on hitting a goal was not my focus.
I would later get to know Chely quite well through many meetings from various events and concerts. I thanked her

and relayed this story of how much her small amount of time shared had meant to my mom, and she was very surprised. As I recall, she was really surprised not knowing how to respond and was very touched by how she had unknowingly helped someone.

A few weeks after we were back at our home, Mom told me that these people have many of the same things we do. She then said she really would like to go home now. I tried to explain to her that we were home. It was after this confusing conversation that things finally clicked with me: we had a serious problem.

A few evenings after I returned from work, I found Mom standing beside her car with the rear passenger door open. She looked rather angry and frustrated. It turns out that she believed my niece, Christy, was sitting in the car and refusing to get out. She could not understand why Christy would not listen to her and step out of the car.

I once walked into the living room and was told that a little girl was sitting on the edge of the coffee table smiling at her. Mom wondered what the girl's name was and why she was on the table. She was afraid the girl would fall off the table and hurt herself. I did something rather stupid and walked over to the edge of the table and pushed out my hand to show there was no one there. This was a big mistake. Mom was afraid I had hurt the little girl, and suddenly I realized just how real these hallucinations were to her. I would have paid anything to take those actions back.

A little later one afternoon she said, "Your dad has been at the store for a long time. I'm afraid he might get lost in that big store. Maybe I should call and have them check on him." I then had to do a very difficult thing. I said, "Mom, you know Dad passed away three years ago." She broke down in tears and said, "Yes, I know." I comforted her for a while, not really knowing what to do or say. Knowing that she would be able to forget something like this was very much indication things were getting worse. Words cannot describe what I felt.

I am unable to ever recall a time in my life where I felt more unsettled and unsure. The reality of the situation was becoming much clearer, and frankly it left me very confused and scared. Still, there was no thought in my mind that she was going to get much worse. I guess my mind was subconsciously blocking out any possibility that she was dealing with a serious mental condition.

Mom's confusion came more often and not just after sleeping. Also, she began to imagine people and things that were not there. I had already been working overtime to help pay for her medicine and debts, and my debts as well. Her doctor had diagnosed her with early stages of dementia, and the medication for this was very expensive. There was little help from any sources such as insurance, Medicaid, or Medicare. More time at work meant less time to be home to take care of my mother.

My sisters both worked and had no way to be there either. We could not leave her at home alone, so now we were faced with a problem. Even though the President had enacted the Family Medical Leave Act, my employer seemed to not want to allow me anytime off work; in fact, it seemed they wanted to work me even more. I was rarely able to keep my day off and would end up having to work. This just added to our problems.

I was already not getting very much sleep. Mom would wake up several times during the night, and once awake she thought she had slept all night. It didn't matter if she had been in bed five minutes or five hours, she was wide awake once she woke up. I quickly learned that for me to get any rest at all, I had better go to bed when she did, because I had no idea how long she would sleep.

Many nights she would wake up at 3a.m. thinking she needed to iron my uniform for work. I didn't care if it was ironed or not, but she insisted the uniform needed to be ironed.

Things were really beginning to take their toll on me. I was not sleeping, and I was overworked and spending every available moment taking care of my mother. I was getting help on the weekends from my sisters, and a little help during the week from one sister, since she lived close. I was still becoming overwhelmed even with the help they were able to offer. I was the primary caregiver, and that is an around-the-clock role. It does not matter what you try, there is no avoiding the fact you are basically on call 24–7.

I would love to tell you I had the perfect plan for dealing with this, a magic solution that made everything just go away. The truth is that I have no idea how I kept going. I was honestly just hanging on by a thread.

I was able to take a step back and get an idea of what was beginning to transpire.

  This was becoming an obvious role reversal. Things had gone from a parent rearing a child to the child taking care of the parent's every need. The biggest difference is that instead of things getting easier as when a child learns to do things for himself, things get more and more difficult as the parent only regresses with this disease. Instead of them learning to do more things for themselves as a child does, they lose the ability to do even simple things. A parent will celebrate a child's progress, yet in this situation the child celebrates that the parent can still perform basic activities and wonders just how long this will continue to be true. When an adult begins wearing diapers and the caregiver becomes responsible for keeping a clean one on them, then you can learn to truly appreciate everything the parent has done over the years to take care of a child when they were helpless.

  I was at a point where this truth had come home. I knew my parents loved me and had taken care of me during the years as I developed into an adult. I just never realized how much sacrifice and love had gone into that. Fortunately, I was able to look at the current situation and feel it was only right that I take care of my mother in her time of need. After all, she had taken care of me when I needed it. I'm sure she never complained about changing dirty diapers or caring for me when I was sick. She would have just said she loved me, and it was part of the job. Now, it was time to return the favor. I never dreamed I would ever be in the position of having to feed, clothe, and change diapers for one of my parents, yet suddenly that had become my life. Thinking of it now being just a part of my role made it much easier.

As things were becoming worse, I begin to feel I was not measuring up to my role. It felt as if I was failing in my role as caregiver. With the lack of sleep, increased pressure on myself, constant giving of myself, and trying to maintain a somewhat normal life, I was getting dangerously close to having a complete mental, spiritual, emotional, and physical breakdown. I honestly think only God kept me from that point.

Another blessing I received was when one of Mom's friends from church volunteered to pick her up on Sunday mornings. Katherine Tate would come by each week and take her to church and bring her home. Although I do not recommend ever skipping church, this gave me one of my only small times of peace. That alone time became very precious to me, and I'm very thankful for having it. That might have even been just enough of a break to keep me sane.

I know it sounds strange to say that sometimes it is okay to not attend church. Remember, the church is not a building; it is the group of people that meets inside. God has a way of teaching us things outside the walls of the church that we otherwise would miss by sitting in a pew. We don't earn salvation or get any extra credit by attending church. I was learning to be more like Christ by the role I was in. These were valuable lessons that I could and would use later in my life.

One Sunday morning around 8a.m., I awoke to the smell of barbequed chicken. I at first thought how nice it smelled; then I quickly realized Mom was already making lunch! I walked into the kitchen just as she was setting

the table with mashed potatoes, barbequed chicken, homemade biscuits, and creamed corn. I also saw a nice glass of sweet tea. I questioned her as to why we had lunch ready before church. She said we always have our lunch after we get home from church. I knew there was no convincing her that we had not already been to church and that it was time for breakfast and not lunch. I enjoyed an unusual breakfast menu that morning. I was following some wonderful advice we had been given earlier that basically said, "Do not argue with a dementia patient; just go with the fl ow and they will respond much better." How she could still prepare such delicious meals is beyond me. Katherine arrived about an hour later to pick up Mom, but I was not sure if she was going or not. Mom did end up going with her, although I'm sure the smell of barbeque sauce in the air had to make Katherine wonder why we were eating so early. These types of days became the norm around our home.

Another thing keeping me on my toes was the fact that now I had no clue what "role" I was supposed to be playing each day. Let me explain. In her mind, different eras of her life were now coexisting. Simply put, when she saw me, she might be seeing her father, her husband, me, or my brother. I had to be able to quickly switch to whichever person she thought she was seeing, for a wrong response could cause a fit of anger. Lucid moments came and went, and there was no way to know how long they would last. The not knowing if this time the lucid moments might not return can become extremely frustrating.

One evening I had made Manwiches and was eating two of them. She watched me eat them and called me a pig because I had eaten both and not left one for Roger. Obviously, she was seeing me as my father. A few times I would come home from work, and when I walked into my room, I would see a plate with a grilled cheese sandwich on my bed and a glass of Sun Drop with melted ice on the nightstand. I asked about this, and she would either reply that I had asked for the grilled cheese, or that "he" was going to eat it. At this point, I could be seen as any number of people, and sometimes she could be thinking I was there along with one or more of the others I was supposed to be. Once, out of nowhere it seems, she told me, "You know you have two sons." She said it with conviction and anger. Obviously, she thought she was talking to my father instead of to me. I had to wonder though, exactly what she was trying to say. My brother and I were never alive at the same time, so this completely confused me as to what she might have been talking about.

All too often this was how my evenings after work would go. It is amazing to me when I look back on this time, that I did not completely lose it. I honestly do not know how I was able to perform my duties at workday in and day out. Maybe the one-hour drive each way was enough to help me regroup. One thing I began to count on each night as I drove home was to begin slowing down as I topped the hill where our church sat. Many times, I would find Mom sitting there outside on the steps waiting for church to begin. She did not realize it was not church night and could not understand why no one would inform her of a change in the schedule. I know it was ingrained in her that her place was at church whenever those doors were open. She knew her place was in the house of God. Before she

got too confused, every morning and every evening I could see her sitting at the kitchen table reading her Bible. She knew what mattered in life, and this was evident by me knowing where she would be each evening on my way home from work.

I mentioned earlier that things had gotten way too complicated for my sisters and me to be able to care for her by ourselves. We were able to locate an adult daycare, and this seemed to be the perfect answer to our problem. This would give us peace of mind that she had great care during the day, and we would be able to take care of her at night. Weekends, my sisters could rotate turns watching her as I worked.

One morning I was putting her coat on her, and we were waiting for the bus to pick her up. I asked if she knew who I was and what we were doing. She smiled and said, "You are my daddy, and we are waiting for the school bus to arrive." We were waiting for my sister to stop by. Since I had to be at work before the bus would arrive, she would come by and wait with Mom until the bus picked her up. She would always call Janet by the name of Louise. So, in her mind I was her father, and my sister was her sister.

If you are having trouble at this point keeping up with who is supposed to be who and just who they really are, try living this day in and day out. It is amazing how the human brain can become so confused so quickly. It is also very sad to watch as a person deteriorates mentally right before your eyes.

Well, the perfect solution did not last very long. It became apparent that she was declining too quickly for the adult daycare to be able to allow us to continue to let her go there. She was approaching a point of being beyond their point of care. I'm thinking, *beyond their point of care. How about our point of care*? We had been taking care of her for several years and we are untrained, yet someone who is trained could not take care of her? I guess you can see just why we were becoming frustrated.

Making matters worse we had to wonder just how closely she was being monitored. She was coming home with minor injuries and bruises almost daily at this point. As usual in these types of scenarios, there is always an "explanation" as to what transpired. We will never know if these were just accidents or the result of neglect.

A very sad event was the day she came home with chocolate ice cream all over the front of her shirt. I questioned her as to how the chocolate got onto her clothes and she said she had dropped it and they refused to give her another one. Imagine how heartbroken I was at the thought of her thinking she was getting a tasty treat only to have it slip from her hand. Even worse, knowing she could not receive a replacement for that one. It's all I can do to type these words without taking a break to wipe away tears.

Now we had a new problem. If the adult daycare was no longer an option, what could we do? None of us three children were able to be able to leave work to care for her. None of us had the luxury of being able to take a leave of absence, and the Family Medical Leave Act was being completely ignored by my company, so I could not use my combined sick leave and annual leave to care for my mom. Even if we did have the opportunity to take some time off, it would still just be a temporary solution.

We now were down to only two choices. We could hire someone to live in and be a paid caregiver, or we could search for an assisted-living home. Neither option was a choice we wanted to make. Unfortunately, hiring a nurse to live in the home was just way too expensive for any of us to be able to handle. That left us with the worst-case scenario: we would have to place her in an assisted-living home. Trust me, when you reach this decision, it is one of the most difficult and painful things you will ever have to face. I hope no one reading this ever experiences going through that gut wrenching decision.

Chapter 5

NURSING HOME: FIRST CHRISTMAS MIRACLE

By the fall of 1998, it was apparent we could no longer offer Mom the care she required. I had been primary caregiver for over two years and greatly appreciated the help offered by my sisters and a few close family friends. In the end, it was just not enough. We were not qualified to deliver the type of around-the-clock care now needed.

We had enrolled her in an adult daycare in the summer; however, now just a few months later, she was beyond their level of care as well. This nasty disease was ravaging through her mind rapidly. It was so heart wrenching seeing such a beautiful mind laid to waste so quickly.

The thoughts of losing the ability to do anything at all for yourself are unnerving. There are no words to adequately express the feelings of seeing it played out before your very eyes in someone you love. "Helpless" is an inadequate description of watching something as brilliant and complex as the human mind turn to mush.

When we began the search for an assisted-living facility to place our mother in, this was the worst feeling I have ever experienced. Many years ago, she had asked that no matter what happened, to never be placed in a nursing home. Feelings of total failure and betrayal were flooding my head.

I knew in my heart this was the only option we had left, yet it still felt as if someone had reached into my chest and ripped out my heart.

I was already mentally, physically, spiritually, and emotionally spent. I fully realized the task at hand would be even more draining. I was completely surprised how few facilities existed that had "locked units" to handle people in this condition. Finding a facility with an opening for a new patient is like looking for Waldo.

We learned of a place about a two-hour drive away that currently had an opening. We went to visit and found the location quite charming. It was in the mountains and located very near a lake. This would have made a nice setting for a weekend getaway or vacation. We interviewed with management and staff. It seemed that maybe this place would work. The only problem was we felt it was too far away. This would drastically limit the number of times per week we could visit and the length of the visits as well.

We still had some medical tests to go through as required by state law. After getting the TB results back, the nurse jokingly said, "Well I guess we don't have to keep you." My mom replied, "Thank you, thank you, thank you!" The poor nurse looked as if she would burst into tears. I mustered as much of a smile as I could to reassure her, and we went to make payment arrangements.

Irony would prevail as the date for us to move Mom into her new home would be February 14, 1999. What are the odds? The day most Americans celebrate as a day of love, we are placing our mother in an assisted-living home. This felt like anything other than love. At least it wasn't Mother's Day. The saddest part was the thought that we would be sneaking out of the building as she was being shown areas of her new home.

The ride back was odd to say the least. We were all very quiet, and most attempts at conversation were rather awkward. We did manage to have some meaningless chatter that helped pass the time. Any distraction was good for us. What are you supposed to say, and what are you supposed to feel?

I had never felt so alone in all my life as I did the evening I returned to our home. This should have been the first night in years I would be able to sleep the entire night without having to worry or listen for Mom to get up. Sleep was one of the last things on my mind. I had been through an unexpected, devastating breakup and divorce almost exactly five years prior, and that pain was nothing compared to the emptiness I now felt inside.

I'm sure I wore paths in the carpet as I walked from room to room. I even felt a strong sense of fear, as in the kind of fear when you return home to an empty dark house. That is how my soul felt empty and dark. I felt angry, scared, devastated, and tremendously guilty. I know there is nothing wrong with placing a loved one into a facility that offers them the medical care and security they require, yet until you are faced with this decision you can never understand the full impact of the reality of when you do it.

So many memories, good and bad, flooded my mind. I am so surprised I had not already had a complete emotional, mental, or physical breakdown. I know beyond a shadow of a doubt, unless I am Superman, it was the grace and love of God that carried me through those past few years. I could appreciate all the lessons I had learned from the divorce, financial stress, and my father's death. It is true that God will never allow us to endure any test that we cannot get through, and He will provide a way out. He will allow us to be pushed beyond our limits though, so He can walk us through. I, however, felt anything other than sure at that moment.

The way out is much more like walking us through it. Character is built during pain and difficult times much like fire purges flaws in gold and purifies the metal. The analogy of a ship has been used many times. A ship being built in a shipyard looks nice. As it is towed out of the harbor, it appears to be a majestic vessel; however, until it is out at sea and a storm tosses it around in rough water, there is no way to know if it is truly seaworthy.

I was experiencing some rough waters, and yet I was not aware of the testing I was currently facing. I was living hour by hour, and my goal was surviving from one to the next. I would not realize until later just how each storm was making me better prepared to face the bigger storms in my life. It is much like the fact that every person's life is a story, yet we do not know we are in a story as it is unfolding. Many things and people play a role in our story, and thus will shape our lives and the story or legacy we leave behind.

The empty house no longer felt like a home; it was no more than an empty shell. My heart understood that well since it was just as empty. I didn't even want to entertain the thoughts of work the next morning and having to be nice to coworkers and customers. Honestly, I was not feeling like being nice to anyone or anything. This included myself, just let me hide.

I went outside to visit and feed my two dogs. My babies were all I had at this point. Mamie and Dillon, (a Dalmatian and golden retriever) were there to eagerly greet me. I could at least take care of their needs without feeling like a total screw-up. Dillon was probably the coolest pet I have ever had. Golden Retrievers are known to be very affectionate. He knew he was loved and always gave a running, jumping hug whether you wanted it or not. I recalled my mom telling me once about how obvious his love was for me, by how different he acted when I was around. Mamie was not as affectionate as Dillon; still she was a loving pet as well. She was getting a little age on her and a little more set in her ways. I was able to get into a better frame of mind by spending times with my dogs.

One of my stress releases the past few years had been to shoot basketball on a portable goal I had set up in the backyard. Many times, my mom would come out to play a game that I began calling "way to go man." Anytime I made a shot, she would yell "way to go man." I found myself chuckling as I took a few halfhearted shots that night I could still hear her saying that. In my mind, I was thinking *yeah way to go man, you just abandoned your mom.*

 I have often heard it said that it is darkest before the dawn, and that was a long dark night. It felt very strange to wake up to an empty house. It was as if the house had lost its spirit. That place was never the same when she was absent; even in her reduced mental state, there was some kind of extra life she added to the house. It had always been that way. Even my dad thought the same when he was still alive. The moment Mom pulled into the driveway or walked through the door; things changed. Now that agent of change would never again walk through the door. Suddenly that home would forever be just a house, its soul and spirit had vanished.

 I have no recollection of how work went the Monday after we took Mom to the facility. I know I went, and I know I returned home anything else is lost to me. Getting some type of normal life going again was not so easy. One thing that helped was that I had found a set of left-handed golf clubs a few months before and would go with my friends Jeff and Mike to a par-3 course and take some frustration out on a few innocent golf balls. It was during this time that I hit my first and only hole-in–one. Did I ever need that miracle shot! My friends were as shocked as I was when that little white ball fell into the cup. I was only trying to hit it hard enough to clear a water hazard and created a miracle shot. That memory made me realize that life can also be that way. We are just struggling through, then reach inside with all our strength to clear a hurdle or obstacle and don't even realize we were walking straight into a miracle.

This would be followed most weeks by a trip to visit my mom. These weekday visits were very short as compared to visits on Sunday. Mom was still very active and would constantly walk the halls; I could not even begin to tell you how many miles we covered in those visits. I think the staff was thrilled to see me so they would not have to walk with her. There was very little communication as the damage to her mind was rapidly increasing. The last thing to go was her mobility, and I believe much of that was medically induced so they could keep a better eye on her.

Several incidents happened, and we were very disturbed. After having thought we had found a good place that would take excellent care of Mom, we had to question that and eventually find another place for her to live. We received word that she had fallen and broken her collarbone. She had already been to the doctor and had it taken care of. Mom had always been extremely healthy, never having been in the hospital other than for two miscarriages and the birth of four children. The only time she had ever been sick was a few times with the fl u and an occasional migraine headache that she called the "sick headache" because of how it forced her to bed for the day. We really didn't think too much about the fall; after all, we thought with less sense of balance and medication, a fall was bound to happen.

A few weeks later, we had a terrible shock. The manager of the facility called my sister to inform her that Mom had been hit by another patient and had some slight bruising.

They had assured us she had been to the doctor, and everything was fi ne. We went to visit her and were totally shocked at what we saw. One entire side of her face was blue, purple, and red. It looked as if she had been beaten, not punched, or hit. We had tremendous doubt as to an elderly man with Alzheimer's being able to inflict this type of damage.

We wanted answers, and of course this incident had happened outside the view of the video cameras. There was no way to know what had taken place. We were in a definite catch-22 at this point. If we left her there, we would be fearful for her safety; if we removed her, we had no place to take her. We informed the staff that we were removing her as soon as we located another place with an opening. In the meantime, some relatives, and friends (who meant well) informed social services of this incident, and an investigation was launched. Fortunately, we had already begun the process of locating a new location. We appreciated those who cared so much for Mom's safety, yet they put our backs against the wall. Due to being investigated, the facility gave us an evacuation date. This was unreal. We were not only faced with worrying about what type of care she was receiving; it was now a time issue as well. Seemed as if we were being punished from all sides at once.

There is no way to even begin to describe the jumbled mess my thoughts and brain were in at this point. I wanted to be angry at someone, yet there was no evidence of who to direct the anger. "Helpless, frustrated, and completely uncertain" would be an understatement. It felt as if things just kept going from bad to worse. I was not able to go to church as much at this point due to the length of the drive for visiting my mom. I was still able to hold onto my faith in God, although at times it was wearing rather thin. Somehow, probably only through a miracle, I was not angry at those involved in the incident. I was angry that this was allowed to happen, and questioned how it could have happened. The anger I had could not be directed at anyone, and somehow the Lord allowed me to forgive those involved. This was not instant and not easy. Part of me wanted very much to inflict as much harm as humanly possible on the staff member that we suspected was truly responsible; yet somehow, someway God got through to me that a reaction such as that would do no one any good. I eventually, was able to let the anger go and only had the thoughts of letting my mom down once again to deal with. It seemed no matter what we did, it was always the wrong move.

  Honestly, I was not sure there would be any right or wrong moves. This situation turned out to be a blessing in disguise. We located a newer facility within a few miles of my sister Bobbie's home. We were able to move our mother and relax in the peace that she was now out of danger from anymore "accidents." This was a good move for everyone, especially knowing we were close enough that we could keep a better eye on the care that she was receiving.

The Christmas season of 2001 would hold in store an unforgettable event for me. Christmas day, my sister Bobbie hosted our family dinner at her home. We met for lunch and had family time for the early afternoon hours. I had already decided I would leave early and stop by to see my mom. She had not been able to communicate with us for quite some time, and she was also in a wheelchair at that point. A visit was sometimes rewarded by a faint trace of a smile or a tighter grip on your hand, nothing really of much notice. I had been somewhat depressed during the Christmas season, and I wanted to visit my mother. I felt there was no real reason to visit her on Christmas day other than to know that I did spend time with her on this day. I had been praying for several weeks okay, maybe begging is more accurate that I would be able to have some sort of recognition from her, even if only for a second. I was asking for anything that would let me know she knew I was there or that she still recognized me. By this point, to us, it felt she was no longer there—only her body. We had no way to know how much of her mind was still working. I believe that the unknown is one of the toughest parts to deal with. There is no way, once communication is gone, to know what is going on in the person's mind.

I said my same prayer one more time: that Mom would show me somehow that she did, in fact, know I was there. I really don't think I was putting much faith in the fact I would get an answer. I only wanted a second of clarity from her, nothing more. I so wanted to just have real contact with her again.

We sat in the parlor, and several other residents were watching basketball on TV. A couple was there together both having a conversation; however, each conversation was to themselves, not to the other person. I was thinking this was feeling like anything but Christmas. I tried to have some form of conversation and felt as if nothing I said was getting through.

It was getting close to the time I had planned to leave, so just for fun I thought I would try something. Guess I was just trying to amuse myself or keep my sanity or both. Anyway, we used to play a little game when we would hug sometimes. Basically, we would hug, then at an unexpected time, one would blow into the other's ear and he or she would respond by pretending to smack bubble gum and say, "I love you, baby." We had seen that in a movie many years before. We thought it humorous that the actor had gum in his mouth during what was supposed to be a serious love scene. It had become a running joke with us from then on. So, that day I gave her a hug and blew into her ear and I was *shocked* when she turned her head slightly and blew back into my ear. Her memory and recognition were mostly 99.9 percent gone at that point, and yet she somehow remembered how to respond to our little game.

I just sat there in disbelief. Did that just happen? I had not only been granted my request for her to have a second of clarity, but I had no doubt that at that moment she did know me and what I was attempting to do. My prayer had been not only answered but answered in dramatic fashion as to leave no doubt in my mind. A Christmas miracle to say the least!

It reminded me of how we pray for things, and most of the time we never really have any faith that the prayer will be answered. It is almost as if we are saying that whatever we are praying about is too big or too difficult for God to handle. Sometimes it takes a little reminder that, yes, He hears us and, yes, He can handle anything if He so chooses. So many times, when we see or hear of God doing something great, we'll ask a question such as, can you believe God did that? This is rather comical, when you consider that we question a prayer being answered in a marvelous way, yet accept that He created the universe, caused a virgin birth, and resurrected His Son, Jesus, from the dead. He did all that, yet why are we surprised when a prayer is answered? That's why we are human: He is God, and we are not.

What really amazes me is that He will feel compassion and answer even the smallest of things. We seem to forget that He loves us enough to do even those small things for us.

I must admit, I was in awe of what had happened. I believe that up until this page is being read that I had not shared this with more than six or seven people. I wanted to make sure it was told in context, so as not to distort its full meaning.

Chapter Six

~

THE MOVE

In 1996, I had begun to travel to many areas of the country with a small group of friends to see concerts. We had originally met on fan sites of the artists that we were following. Most of the time, we would meet in Nashville due to its central location to our home bases and concert sites.

Many members of the group developed strong friendships, and it didn't take very long for Nashville to become second home for many of us. We would usually room together during Fan Fair each summer in Nashville. A few had begun to talk about moving there, since that's where we spent most of our free time anyway.

During the drive from Texas to Alabama with my friend Michelle, we seriously began to discuss moving to Nashville along with a yet-to-be--determined third roommate. This was in early 2000, and my mother was no longer recognizing anyone, so I thought maybe that would be a good time for a change and to just get away for a while. I was fortunate enough to work for one of the nation's largest employers, so I basically could transfer to any city in the country.

I submitted paperwork for a mutual job swap and for a transfer. The difference being a mutual swap meant I would stay full-time and just trade cities with another employee, and a transfer would mean I would be part-time flexible for a short while.

As time went on, I began to feel that Nashville would indeed become my home, although the process of changing locations seemed to be going nowhere. I still could not shake the feeling of a strong pull to that city Months turned into years, and it seemed there would be no way for me to make the move. I was content with working in Charlotte, and I loved the Hornets and the Panthers, so no worries if I had to stay in North Carolina. I enjoyed my coworkers and had some friends on my route at work as well.

Late January or early February 2002, I received a letter from Nashville informing me they had an opening if I was still interested in a transfer. I decided to give it a try, and after returning the enclosed paperwork, I was notified just a few weeks later that everything had been approved.

I had mixed emotions about leaving for a new state; however, I had an inner peace about beginning a new life somewhere else. I also had the feeling that there was more to this move, that I was being drawn to this city for a much deeper reason. That would not be known to me for over another year, and not fully realized until another year or so after that time.

Things happened so fast with the transfer being finalized that I went to work in Nashville before actually moving there. I reported to work there and took a few days of vacation after the first week in order to move my belongings.

Moving to a new state, beginning work with a new office, and basically knowing only two people who lived in the entire state was not easy. There were days when I wondered if I had made a wise decision. I knew I had an eighteen-month commitment, so I was willing to give it a shot and see what happened.

I was also wondering if I was abandoning my mother. I quickly realized that visiting every few weeks would not be too different from me living in the same state. She would not even know if I was in the room, so that somewhat eased my mind.

At that point, I was in desperate need of a change of scenery, and I needed to remove myself from the constant daily reminders of the past few years. I was working so much that I really had no time to be depressed or to dwell on the negative things of recent memory.

In August, my friend Paul from Ohio brought our friend Kim from Michigan to Brentwood to visit for the weekend. We were planning to visit some shows and hangout for the weekend. We were having an enjoyable time.

The three of us decided on Sunday afternoon to go to Best Buy in Cool Springs to look for a CD that was a new release. I was browsing around as Kim searched for her CD. Paul walked over and asked me if I had ever seen Garth Brooks up close, and I told him that I had not. He said to go on over to the box section and I would see him and Trisha Yearwood. He was right; it was Garth and

Trisha. They picked up a Chris LeDoux boxed set, and a cashier opened a separate register for them.

I decided to walk outside and wait for them to exit. I knew I needed to share a story with Garth, and this might be the only chance I would ever have. Normally, I would not approach a celebrity in that way unless I already knew them, or I was with someone they knew.

As Garth Brooks came my way, I asked him if he had a second so that I could share something with him briefly. He said sure. He introduced himself, shook my hand, and introduced me to Miss Yearwood as he called her. I knew he had lost his mother recently, and I wanted to share with him just how his music and his character had touched my mom's life. His eyes were misty as I told him about us missing him at Fan Fair the year he had signed for thirty-six straight hours, and that we found out the following day he had been there. I shared that she did get a chance to see him in concert; however, the seats were really bad, and she couldn't really see him that well. I noticed a sincere appreciation in his eyes as he heard me talk about how she told everyone to expect great things from him when he was first starting out. Also, I told him how she would sit in front of the TV with her fingers crossed saying, "Please, oh please let it be Garth" when he was up for an award, and how she would be thrilled with each of his wins. I concluded with sharing just how much "If Tomorrow Never Comes" had meant to her just before my father's death and how living out that song had made those last days together more bearable.

I had already mentioned the background of her battle with Alzheimer's, and that she was now in a nursing home. Hearing that two of the people she had always wanted to meet were Conway Twitty and him, Garth looked at his watch, then at Trisha, and as she nodded, he asked which facility Mom was in. I informed him she was in North Carolina, and he said, "Oh." It took a minute for it to register with me: I was standing there chatting with the current biggest name in the music business, and he was going to take a few moments to stop by and see my mother had she been in the area. He said, "Well, next time you are visiting her, after you give her the hug you are going to give her, give her one from me." He stated he meant it and wanted me to tell her. He had even asked her name.

The only reason I relate this story here is to acknowledge that when two humans share a similar painful experience, it is easy to understand. There is an instant bond formed. Also, I wanted to take the opportunity to publicly thank Garth and Trisha for their kindness and unselfish act in even considering visiting a complete stranger. I will forever appreciate seeing the sympathy and compassion in the eyes of Garth Brooks as he heard about this little lady. Also, I feel it shows just how the events written about in this book can impact the lives of those who hear them.

Tragedy and death are great equalizers. When two people share a similar experience of loss or pain, no longer will social and economic status matter, nor will ethnic or geographical backgrounds. A parking lot in Brentwood, Tennessee served as a place where this truth would play out. Three individuals from completely different walks of life stood and shared a moment that words will never describe. One had already lost his mother, and the other would soon lose his.

Ironically, many people I know would have given anything for this experience. They would have been completely clueless as to what was really happening. I felt sad, guilty, and depressed. I had just spent about fifteen minutes in meaningful conversation with one of the few people my mother truly wished to meet. I would have given anything in that moment to have been able to have her there with us. It seemed rather unfair for me to have the experience she had so dearly longed to have. Fortunately, the moment was not lost on me. I knew that it was an opportunity to share about someone who was special to me with someone that she admired, and personally pass along the impact that his life's work had on someone. I know that as an artist, that means as much many times as awards or CD sales. So, to Garth Brooks, THANK YOU!

The early weeks of the move were rather rough, but I quickly adjusted. In November 2002, I found a new church, Brentwood Baptist Church, and would begin to make a new circle of friends. I was not seeing my music friends quite as much due to my work and changes in each of our life directions.

BBC offered a Friday night service that was a scaled-down, more casual version of the Sunday service. I began to go to this service and found a singles group that had a Bible study class that met on the same night. The group would go out for dinner after the service, and this allowed me a chance to make new friends, some who would prove to be valued friends in the future.

  Distancing myself from "home" and making new, quality friends provided a much-needed change of pace for me. I began to regroup mentally in a sense. It is difficult to realize just how much of yourself you have lost until you are able to stop and step back. I was finally beginning to recover some lost social skills and get back into the game of life.

Chapter Seven

~

THE CALL: GOING HOME

Christmas season 2002 had rolled around, and I was facing something I have never had to deal with before: working on Christmas day. This was a prospect I had never even wanted to think about doing. My first Christmas in Tennessee and first away from my family, and I would be working. This was not the way I had hoped things would work out for the season.

The Sunday night movie about two weeks before Christmas was *The Christmas Shoes*. I taped the movie, knowing it might be difficult to watch it straight through. I tried to watch the movie, but it was just too close to home for me. The entire time, I could not shake the feeling that my mom would die at Christmas too. I kept having that "I've got to get home for Christmas" feeling. I knew this was impossible since I would be working on Christmas day. It finally took me three or four days to finish watching the movie.

The Friday before Christmas, I am covered up at work. I was sitting on 17th Ave. South, a part of Music Row, trying to organize the parcels I will be delivering for that street when my cell phone rang. I noticed on the caller ID that it was from a 704-area code, and in my mind, this could only mean bad news. The call was from my oldest sister telling me they had to take my mother to the emergency room a few times earlier in the week and that her vitals were just not right. She said that I might want to make arrangements to get home. Before I could even process what I had just heard, she called back a few minutes later with an update: we were probably looking at just a few more days at most before our mother passed away.

A coworker showed up to help me out with the rest of the route. After making it back to the office a few hours later, I told my manager about the calls and that I needed to make a trip to North Carolina. His response was, "I only have one question. What are you still doing here? You only have one mother, so go home and we'll worry about covering the route."

I went to my apartment and when I checked my mail, I had an unexpected Christmas card from my leasing agent, Crystal. We had become close friends, and I was hoping to actually take her out soon. Anyway, she had left me a very sweet thank-you note for being there for her and for all the ways I had helped her. Needless to say, this note could not have come to me at a better time. The perfect words from the right person, at just the right time. I began to grab a few things and tried to pack. I soon realized I was way too exhausted to make the 420-mile drive back to North Carolina that night. I called to make sure I would be able to have time to make it if I waited until Saturday morning to leave. The report I got was that things had slightly improved somewhat, so that made me feel a little less urgency. I knew there was no way I would be alert enough to make that drive through the mountains, so instead of starting out right away, I made a few calls to arrange for a place to stay and took care of a few other details.

Saturday morning, I headed out before sunrise to ensure I could get into town as early as possible. During the drive, I heard the song *"The Baby"* by Blake Shelton for the first time. I was thinking, *Man this really sounds very close to an idea I have for a song.* I was able to closely relate to the character in the song. The words jumped out at me when he sang about driving to see his dying mother and not being able to get there in time. All I could think was, *what if this happens to me?*

There were so many emotions and thoughts going through my mind as I drove what seemed more like seven days than seven hours. I finally made it back, and I checked in as soon as I could to get the latest update. It appeared that the worst might be over for now. After this, I went to the nursing center to visit my mother, and honestly, I could not see very much difference from when I was last home a few months prior to this visit.

Naturally, I was relieved to have made it with time to spare. This was not the type of visit I wanted to make, knowing I would be in town until she passed away.

How do you wrap your mind around the fact that the only way you are going to end this visit and return home is after the death of someone very close to you? It is really strange to have so much time to think about the fact that someone whom you love and have known your entire life is going to die at any time. The fact is that, for our immediate family, it seems as if our mother had already died several years ago due to the devastation of the disease. Now, we were preparing our minds for the realization that soon she was going to cease to exist in any form. So many thoughts, feelings, and emotions just seemed to flood my mind. There were just too many things to try to process. The human brain is a fascinating mechanism, and the most amazing function, in my opinion, is its ability to shut down certain areas to safeguard against a mental overload.

Chapter Eight

~

DAYS BY HER SIDE: REFLECTIONS AND THOUGHTS

Sitting beside a parent's hospital bed, not knowing if she even knows you are in the room, can be very disturbing. I didn't mind spending time with my mother; I just wished I knew if she was aware I was there, and if she knew who I was. It had been so long since any communication was possible. I held out the hope that somewhere deep in her mind she could recognize my voice as I talked with her.

The main thing I thought about was that Alzheimer's and dementia are the cruelest diseases anyone could ever have to endure. It is heartbreaking to see a person, especially someone you love dearly, mentally regress. By this point, my mother was just a shell of her former self, the once warm, loving eyes now yellow and glazed. It was almost as if her soul were now gone.

I felt so helpless to see her only existence being to just lie there. Naturally, the Why? questions begin to surface. Why did someone so sweet and so caring need to endure such a horrible and humiliating disease? Why does nothing like this ever seem to happen to the really bad people of the world? Why did this happen to her at such an early age? Why did it take so little time for her to deteriorate to this point? There were no answers. I knew deep in my heart that God had some purpose in allowing this to happen to her. I had no clue what that could possibly be, yet understood it had to be true.

I had to be brutally honest with myself at this point. Nothing seemed fair. Yeah, I questioned God; and I asked all of the why questions. The real question was, *can I handle His answers*? I could see no way good could come out of this, until I really was willing to put my emotions and desires aside and take an honest look at how things might play out.

After about three days, I begin to wonder if we had been misinformed. It appeared there were no changes in her condition. I called back to work to update them as best I could. At this point, I begin to have a battle raging inside of me. I was torn between deciding if I would stay there for who knows how long or if I would return to Tennessee and then come back to North Carolina again when things took a turn for the worse.

I was thinking, *alright, what if I stay for two or three weeks, and she is still the same*? I would have missed work and then possibly have to return here as soon as I got back to Tennessee. Then I began to wonder, *what if I decide to go back home, then get a call that she has passed away during my travel?*

After much thought and prayer, I felt a peace that I was right where I needed to be. I determined that I would stay as long as I was needed. If it dragged out for very long, my work would not be happy, but they would just have to get over it. Basically, we kept a family member by Mom's side 24–7. We had no clue how much time she had left, and we wanted someone to be there to alert the rest of us if we needed to get there on a minute's notice. I don't really think any of us got much rest or sleep during this time.

I thought how ironic it was that I didn't have to work on Christmas day after all. It was as if she had sensed that and made sure I would be able to be home with her for Christmas. We would not spend our first Christmas apart after all.

It is amazing the things you can recall at a time like this. The simplest of remembrances seemed to be a treasured thought. Yes, all the wasted time or missed opportunities tend to surface as well. Unfortunately, I had recalled making a stupid statement that I couldn't wait to move out of her house. At this point, I would have probably given anything to go back in time a few years and relive those wonderful times.

I kept thinking that if I had only known she would be in this condition so quickly, I would have made sure to spend as much time together as possible. I wondered why I had not taken more photographs or videos. All sorts of things spin through the mind. Fortunately, I thought, *I am so thankful for the time I have now to spend with my mother.* I knew if the roles were reversed that she would be spending every possible second with me and not worrying about the past; instead, she would enjoy the time that was left. It is very surreal when the finality of life begins to sink in. Just a few years before, we were traveling together, and now I was sitting beside her.

bed knowing, she would die soon. I would face each day not knowing if this would be our last time to spend together.

The one thing at the back of my mind was my own mortality. I had felt all my life that my purpose in being born was to fill the void left by my brother Steve's death. I knew I was supposed to be there to watch over my mother. That became more apparent after my father's death when I moved in with Mom to take care of her. Now, I can see what a wise move that turned out to be. I could not have known that at the time; however, it was clear now.

So, I was wondering what would happen after she died. Would my mission be complete, and I, too, would pass away? I had no clue. As I said, my mind was spinning, and all sorts of weird thoughts were processing through my brain at this point. Still, I had to wonder what the future held for me after having such a definite role as caregiver, before and during her illness.

I realized that it was not the time to try to deal with such thoughts. I pushed all that out of my mind and focused on enjoying, the best I could, the time left together. That is exactly what I did. I will forever be grateful for those few hours alone. I have no clue how much time passed; however, I would not trade a single second of it for any amount of money.

There was an almost eerie feeling of peace. It is very difficult to capture those moments in time through words. This was one of those times that seem to stand still and nothing whatsoever in the world means anything. The only thing that matters in the moment is taking in every possible second of time and savoring each emotion.

I had never been so focused on doing absolutely nothing other than enjoying the moment. I so wish there were adequate words to describe the scene; however, as clichéd as it sounds, you truly had to be there. Unfortunately, we never seem to take enough time out of our busy lives to just completely shut out the world and enjoy being with our loved ones. There are so many things that can wait, yet it seems we put everything ahead of our friends and family.

The greatest two gifts you can ever give anyone would be your undivided attention and your time. Two things that cost so little, yet we are so unwilling to give. I have no way of ever knowing if my mother knew I was sitting in that room with her or not. What I do know is I took full advantage of the time together to make lasting memories of sharing the gift of time. This was a gift I knew was quickly fading, as time was fleeting. I'm sure this will remain one of my favorite moments of time.

A thought that did occur to me is how we so easily confuse our priorities. We have this insane idea that we need to work ourselves to death to make a few more dollars. In the end, what does this accomplish? The only thing it does is allow us to buy more stuff as if we needed anything else. Honestly, it makes me wonder if we were better off with less technology and a simpler way of life.

Chapter Nine

~

WAL-MART AND SANTA

The night of the twenty-third, a youth group, along with a
Hispanic Santa, came through the hallways singing
Christmas carols. We noticed that Mom was having a slight
response to the music. She had long lost her ability to
communicate and was mostly "just there." We all just
looked at each other and were in awe realizing that she
recognized the music. Any response to anything was
unheard of by now. Imagine us sitting there knowing our
mother could die at any time, and a group of young people
begin to sing "Silent Night." Never before had I truly heard
the words of this song. It was eerie and surreal to take in
how applicable this song was to this scene.

A short time later, Santa came around to visit room to
room. This was the first time I had ever seen a Hispanic
Santa, and that caught my attention. Santa was all cheerful
and jolly until he crossed the doorway to my mother's
room. He stopped, almost frozen in place. His eyes said it
all. One of my spiritual gifts is discernment, and with that I
can read so much into what is in someone's eyes. I had
never seen such heartfelt compassion in the eyes of a
stranger. Immediately to my mind came the verse in
Hebrews, about entertaining angels unaware. Those eyes
would stay with me. It was as if he looked right into the
soul of each of us. Santa looked in his bag, felt around a

little, and then pulled out an angel doll. This might not seem like anything unusual until you know that Mom always believed God provided guardian angels to watch over us. She really believed we encounter angels at various times and that they were always years and enjoyed reading about them and how God used them.

Before she had gotten to the point of needing the care of a nursing facility, I would have to stop on my way home from work to pick her up from church. She would go there almost daily thinking it was church night. She kept wondering why no one had called her to let her know that the service was canceled. My mother may not have known which night to go, but she knew her place was in church, and she was to be there to worship.

After Mom received the angel doll that night, I had to investigate for myself. Something just didn't seem real about the previous scene. I couldn't find Santa. However, I did see that other residents also had their dolls. I began to look in each of the rooms. There were various colors and styles of dolls, but I only saw one other angel doll. It then occurred to me what the odds were of only two angels being given out and that one of them had actually ended up with my mother.

The angel was so appropriate for her, and the timing was perfect. The angel was in her arms constantly from this point on. It was such a sweet picture to see this dear lady lying in bed, holding the angel just as a child holds her doll as she sleeps. She had always talked about how angels held us and protected us, and now she was holding onto an angel in her most trying time. Her face seemed so peaceful as if nothing could harm her.

It was not lost on me what was transpiring; however, it would become much clearer later. You may not be able to fully grasp this scene: a lady who has spent most of her life serving others and being a living witness to holding onto God in the most trying of times was once again showing me how to hold onto God. She had talked so much about how God uses angels to protect and comfort, and now He was showing a very clear picture of this, as my mother was lying on her deathbed holding onto an angel as she awaited death. I honestly think this showed so much how compassionate God is to us.

I went back to the home of my friends, Jamie, and Stephany. They had so graciously allowed me to live with them while I needed to be in North Carolina spending the last days with my mom. They had always been there for me through the years, and now they were more than happy to lend a hand. I tried not to interfere with their daily routine, yet anytime a guest is in your home, things are going to be different. I truly appreciate all they did for me, giving me a place to return to each night to process all that was transpiring.

I continued to think about how the music had invoked a reaction and sense of recognition. I began to feel that we definitely needed to bring some music into her room. At this point, I was exhausted and knew most of the stores were closed or getting ready to close.

The next day was Christmas Eve, and I went to the only retail store in the town: Wal-Mart. I knew I needed to buy a CD player and some music. I was rather stressed inside, wondering if Mom might pass away while I was out shopping for music to play for her. She had always loved music, and Nashville was always a must visit a few times each year. After seeing how she had responded to music the night before, I had to find a way to play some for her. I searched for some compact discs of her favorite artists, but I couldn't find exactly what I was looking for. I did manage to find a few anyway. I had burned (recorded) some compact discs a few nights before I left Tennessee, so those were in my car. I knew I would have enough to play for her.

I still felt a strong urge to get back to the assisted-living center. Quickly gathering all the items that I wanted to purchase, I went to stand in line in the electronics department. There was a better chance of getting out of the store quickly in a department rather than in the regular lines at the front of the store. I was about seven people back in line, and a few others were behind me. I patiently waited there and prayed for the line to move quickly.

Suddenly, a man opened a second register, and no one moved to go over there. If you have ever worked in retail or shopped near Christmas, you know this just does not happen. The fact that no one moved to an open register in and of itself is a miracle. This man looked straight at me and motioned for me to come over. I began to think these people would kill me if I basically left the line to go to the open register. I felt a tap on my shoulder, and an African American lady behind me said, "He opened the register for you. Go!" My head was spinning at this point, and I walked over almost in a trance still, no one else was going to this line. Then a thought almost knocked me down: *What if I only have just enough time to get back to the center before she dies*? I paid for my items and quickly headed for the exit. I did steal a glance back and saw only the one line open and one cashier! My cashier was GONE!! Then I was wondering if I really paid for these items.

Ironically, we ask ourselves if God still performs miracles or speaks to us audibly, then when we experience both, we don't realize it. I have no doubt there were angels that day in the electronics department of that Wal-Mart. I also truly believed God used that lady or was she an angel, to speak to me.

I honestly had to laugh out loud as I walked back to my car. God definitely has a sense of humor. I mean really, would anyone ever expect an angel to be in Wal-Mart? This was just the thing I needed something outrageously ridiculous to laugh about.

I was relieved once I got back to my mother's room and realized all my anxiety had been for nothing. I was happy to see that a family member of the lady on the other side of the room was taking her home for a few days for Christmas. This would mean we would have some privacy.

I played a few songs for Mom: some Christmas, some Christian, Garth, and Conway Twitty. It just so happened that I had some songs I knew she liked on the CDs I had made just a few days earlier. A song that had just been released was "I Can Only Imagine" by MercyMe. I played this one and really listened to the words. It was just the two of us, and I could truly take in what the artist was saying about reaching heaven and meeting Jesus face-to-face. I kept thinking, *Yeah, all I can do is imagine this; however, this wonderful little lady is so very close to living the words of the song.* I took this opportunity to tell her that I loved her and that she was about to receive the greatest Christmas gift anyone could possibly ever get. She ever-so-slightly turned her head. Words could not describe listening to that song and knowing that it was all soon to be a reality for her. I then played "The Dance" by Garth Brooks. A nurse started to walk in, and when she heard that song she had to leave. She later told us that when she opened the door and heard the song playing, knowing what was happening in the room, it was just too much for her to handle.

I had to stop and really be thankful for this time alone. It was a very rare and unexpected opportunity. God had worked so many miracles for us to be together. This was a very special private time and one that I will forever be thankful for being allowed to have. There was no way to know if we would ever again have time alone. All logical thinking seemed to suggest that this would be the last opportunity.

How are you supposed to wrap your mind around the fact that time together with someone you truly love is almost over? I couldn't help but think that if it was not for the promise of eternal life, then this life would be such a tragedy. All the pain and suffering would just be a prelude to more pain and suffering along with separation.

Anyway, it is so sad that we tend to never appreciate time spent with our family and friends until we either lose them or realize we are close to losing them. It would be so much better for each of us if we would realign our priorities and learn to appreciate the truly important things in our lives.

Chapter Ten

~

DYING: ONE LAST CHRISTMAS

I've never really been that much into the gift exchanging or other "normal" aspects of Christmas. Each year after Christmas I would be amazed at all the toys friends and classmates would receive. I thought how rich their families were, when in reality, we were just that poor. I never once thought Santa ripped us off; it all seemed quite normal. Looking back on it, I'm glad it was that way. I can see how we were the rich ones not in money, but in love. I'll probably never know the sacrifices made in order for us to have Christmas each year. My family was close, and we enjoyed the Christmas season, yet each year seemed to lose a little something.

I was working in retail at the time, and seeing how so many people treated this wonderful season and just basically made a mockery out of it really depressed me. I still engaged in the "gift" part of Christmas, giving generously to friends, and not really expecting anything in return. I enjoyed giving! I especially enjoyed the look of surprise and appreciation when giving to an unsuspecting person.

Somewhere along the way, my sisters decided their extended families were getting so big that they couldn't buy presents for everyone. They decided our family would not exchange gifts, so that they would be able to buy for their own families. This shut me out. It was in no way intentional, yet that was the outcome. They had their families to exchange with, and I had me. Don't get me wrong. I completely understood their situation and think they made a wise choice, yet once again Christmas was losing a little more.

I still wanted to celebrate, so I began a tradition on Christmas night with a couple of very close friends and their parents. We would exchange gifts and have dinner. Actually, these friends and I were very much like family to each other. This special celebration would never have happened, had not my former way of celebrating Christmas changed. Now, I had an additional family to celebrate with.

Fast forward to Christmas Day, 2002 when we met for lunch at the home of my oldest sister, Bobbie. I'm not really sure why we met our minds were anywhere but there. We all had the same thought: get back to Mom. We hurriedly went through the motions of Christmas lunch and headed back to visit Mom. I spent most of the day with her. My sisters and their families were doing the same.

It seems each of us had the same secret desire. We just didn't know how to bring it up. We knew it was only a matter of time, as we could see her life slipping away. At one point during the day, I told my mother that she was going to get the most wonderful Christmas gift anyone could imagine. It was my way of letting her know it was okay to go.

Each of us was thinking secretly how wonderful it would be for her to actually be able to meet Jesus face-to-face on Christmas day!! Think about it: the ultimate goal of all Christians is to make it to heaven when we finally leave this world. We didn't want her to die, but we knew she was going to, and we thought how cool it would be if she were able to experience that on Christmas. I guess we thought that would be more appropriate.

We all made the most of the day and enjoyed what we understood would be our last Christmas together as a family. It really brought to reality what Christmas is all about. The presents, tree, lights, and carols are all just fluff. The real joy and experience of Christmas is the love in a family. In a weird way, it was one of the best Christmases we had experienced together. There is no way for me to capture that moment in these pages, nor would I even attempt such a thing. Some experiences are just too special to be understood outside the moment.

On Christmas evening, we thought the time had come. Mom suddenly sat straight up in bed and reached up with one arm as she looked up toward the sky. It appeared she was trying to mouth a few words, and a tear rolled down her face. Then she slowly laid back down, looking almost disappointed. We all felt something, or someone was behind us, but even though we really wanted to look, none of us did. Somehow, we felt we should keep our attention on her. Whatever she had seen, whether real or a vision, was meant for her, and we allowed it to remain that way.

We all decided that we would go home and try to get some rest so we could return early the following morning.

About 3:45a.m. on December 26, 2002, I got a call: I was told that it would not be very long and I should come to the center. When my phone rang, my friends Jamie and Stephany came out of their room, hugged me, and offered the usual condolences. They knew that if my phone rang at that hour, it was time. I rushed over to the nursing home just as it was beginning to sleet.

At around 6:00 a.m., we could tell her shallow breathing had seemed to stop, and we called for a nurse to verify this. Ironically, we thought it was typical of her to have struggled to hang on long enough to not die on Christmas, trying to keep us from having her death to remember each Christmas.

That year we were supposed to all be spending Christmas in different states, and instead we were all together as a family for one last time. It was so clear that this was what Christmas was truly about family! There were no presents, very few reminders that it was even Christmas...yet we had a very special holiday, and I definitely came away with a different perspective. I had always felt there was so much more to Christmas than the typical commercialized, secular celebration that goes on each year. I didn't think I would actually experience the real meaning of Christmas in such an unusual way. What should have been a very difficult and painful memory actually has some important lessons and reminders. I'm able to actually be thankful for all I experienced and learned. I'm very thankful for the additional time we spent together.

Taking time to reflect on those few days and their events, I see that God intended this to be a season of love and family. In the stable that night it was just Mary, Joseph, and the baby Christ when He was first born. Many others would be there later, but for a few moments it was quiet and peaceful. Everything else in the world was of no concern; it was just the little family together. I also have a different perspective on God that night. He had to say good-bye to His Son and would not have Him back in heaven for over thirty-three years…not that time means anything to God. Yet He had to let go in order for others to benefit from His pain.

As Pastor Mike Glenn pointed out a few years ago during a message at Kairos, anytime we see a nativity scene, it should be in the shadow of the cross. Jesus was born for a reason and that was to die. He was to live a perfect and sinless life in order to die in our place. Although the birth is a reason to celebrate, He had a much more important role for being here. Babies are born every day. How often does one grow up to die and then be resurrected after taking on the sin of the entire world? Yes, Jesus came as a man in order to die in man's place.

Reflecting back on the moment of my mother's death, I remember as she slipped away into eternity, she was still tightly holding the angel doll under her arm. The thought struck me as I watched this: *She held the angel as she slept; now the angels are holding her.*

We requested that during the visitation that the angel be placed in her arms. This decision allowed for many opportunities to share some of these stories. Several people commented on the stories and said it should be told, either in song or a book. Finally, that request has been fulfilled.

As a family, we decided instead of one of us keeping the angel, that we would bury it with her. I'm not sure how odd that sounds from the outside; however, we knew it had special meaning.

A few years later, as I reflected more on these events, the following lines came to me:

"Sleeping with the angels.

As they guide her flight

From one realm to the other

Oh, what a precious sight

All through life she shone their light.

Now they hold her tight.

As she's...

Sleeping with the angels

Chapter Eleven

~

FUNERAL THOUGHTS: ANDY RAINES

It is no easy task to plan a funeral, and a funeral a few days after Christmas is even tougher. It seemed that everywhere I turned, I was running into snags concerning one part or the other of getting things in order for the service.

Eventually, everything was completed, and the actual service went extremely well. Mom had always said that when she died, she wanted Rev. Andy Raines to officiate at her service. When we made this request, Andy was available and willing to conduct the service.

Throughout his time as pastor at Mt. Beulah Baptist Church, Andy had always been a shepherding type of pastor. If a member were in the hospital or hurting, he was there. I remember many times when he would return early from a vacation due to a death or sickness of a church member. Andy Raines was truly the definition of loyalty and commitment. I recall my mother saying many times that Andy Raines was not just a pastor, but he was also a friend.

I wish to share a few thoughts that Andy relayed during the funeral service. It was beneficial that Andy had pastored and served with Mom for so many years; it made the service much more personal. The following were points mentioned during her service.

After I had called to inform Andy of Mom's passing, he shared a thought that had occurred to him: Death does not always come as an enemy, but sometimes it comes as a friend by releasing a soul of a diseased body and pain. This was the case in this instance.

Thinking about her life, he related many remembrances of my mother. She had lived a simple life. She was simple in her demeanor: never trying to take the spotlight or be too fl ashy. Simple in her desires: never seeking fortune or fame, satisfied with her life and her friends and family. It didn't take much to make her happy, and she seemed to always be smiling. Simple in her delights: her children and grandchildren brought her much happiness. She loved each of them very much. Mom also took delight in trips and fellowships. Andy mentioned that she enjoyed trips so much, that if the church van was moving, she would be on it. She didn't care so much as to *where* it was going, just that it *was* going.

Fellowships were a chance for her to be with friends and to make new friends. My mother was sincere in her love for family and friends. If her family or friends hurt, she hurt. If they were happy, she joined in their happiness. Friends were as loved as family. She understood that to have a friend you first had to be a friend. Andy made the point that if you were not Ollie's friend, it was not Ollie's fault, because she wanted to be your friend. Her circle of friends was quite large.

She was sure in her Lord and remained steady in faith during peace and pain. Although she faced many hardships throughout her life, Mom never lost sight of who was in charge. At four eleven, she was short in stature, but large in faith she relied on God's power. She always offered hope not criticism and compliments not complaints. Andy said that in his mind, he could still hear her say to him, "Preacher, it's going to be all right; the Lord will take care of you."

For her, church was a place to serve. She came to worship, not just fill a spot on a pew. This was a time for her to fellowship with her Lord and her friends. Church really meant something to her. It was not just a place or a building. It was God's people and a way of life.

Mom was solid in her lessons. She lived what she believed and believed what she lived. Heaven was real to her, and now it is more real than ever. She has been reunited with loved ones and is there awaiting the rest of her family.

Two things are certain: Life is fragile. Death is not concerned with age or social standing. No one can promise that you are going to live; however, you can rest assured that you will die. Unless the Lord returns first, each of us will taste death. No one has ever escaped it, and no one ever will until the return of the Lord.

Chapter Twelve

A DARK TIME: CAREGIVER'S PERSPECTIVE

The caregiver goes through hell! This is no exaggeration, it's the truth put bluntly. Unless you ever walk in those shoes it is next to impossible to grasp any understanding of the inner turmoil that is experienced. The level of stress is off the chart. Couple that with little to no sleep and the result is anger, frustration, and despair. Lifestyles of the patient and the caregiver are dramatically altered. Much soul searching is required, and this goes very deep. A level must be achieved to where a determination is made as to how to continue to live. Unfortunately, in some cases a decision to even live must be faced.

Every single decision will have short-term and long-term effects. Weighing through the potential ramifications only adds more stress. Some of these results are not even realized until it is much too late to correct. Now comes the burden of trying to decide if there was any damage done by something said or some reaction to an event. Living on the edge of a breakdown becomes daily life.

A few of the more common emotions are guilt and the over-all feeling of failure. That feeling of emptiness added to the burden that is already being carried leads to questions of why this happened, how can I make it through, is anyone going to step up and help me. How did things change so quickly? The one question that never goes away is, did I do everything I could or was there more I could have done?

Seeing a stranger that is suffering from Alzheimer's it is easy to just think, *hey look at that crazy old fool*. If you were able to actually know the person before the disease took ahold of their mind, then you can truly understand just how devastating the deterioration can be. It is then that you come to realize they are not crazy old fools after all.

Dementia and Alzheimer's can bring on drastic changes to the person they invade. The memory is not all that changes, there are alterations to the personality, comprehension, and overall thought process. There are so many things that change, many times the patient's actions and reactions are no longer like the person they were before the disease.

A few of the things that I faced were the results of the uncertainty of not knowing what might be discovered in the house. So many things out of the ordinary or just plain strange that would not make sense. I might be walking through the house and discover a potted plant had been mistaken for a toilet. Wash cloths might be in the toilet, leading me to think it was mistaken for the washer. Finding all my mom's socks had been thrown into the dog kennel, never figured that one out. There were even times I had suspected the dry dogfood had been mistakenly eaten as a snack. Just so many things to discover that it became normal to expect the unexpected.

After we had enrolled our mom into a nursing facility, visits could be very stressful. Such a wide range of emotions and questions that would require processing if for no other reason than to help maintain sanity. Sometimes visits would consist of nothing more than sitting there with an arm around her shoulder. We learned to take whatever we could get from the visits. One thing that was always consistent though was the vice like grip on my hand when attempting to leave. Talk about guilt! It was as if she was begging for the visit to not end and her to be left alone.

It was a haunting feeling not knowing what exactly was happening in her mind. Did she have any comprehension? Did she just simply exist and not think anything at all? Maybe her mind was in a constant dream state? Could it have been possible she knew exactly everything that was transpiring around her, yet just find a way to express herself? All these things swirling through your own mind could drive you nuts.

Her blank stare, the look of being a million miles away was unnerving. I had to wonder *did I even exist in that mind.* Was I thought to be someone else? Just exactly what was being processed and how? There was also the possibility that maybe just maybe the raw emotion of genuine love was felt and was enough to bring some comfort and peace to the otherwise chaotic world taking place in her mind. This could explain why she held on for dear life whenever it was time to leave. Maybe she was thinking this was the last time we would ever spend together and would never see each other or spend time together again. Wow, just so many possibilities.

The person suffering with this horrendous disease seems to be tapped in a small corner of their mind. Usually, it is a place in a distant era, a place and time where they felt safe and happy, such as childhood. Is this a coping mechanism used to provide security in facing the fears of the unknown? This time is it consciously chosen or is it just picked as random, sort of by default by the brain?

Reality to the patient is now what is lived out hourly or daily in their minds. Their minds easily, although randomly, slip in and out of the present and past, seemingly with no segue. Almost as if there is a doorway or passage inside their minds they slip through. The "door" opens and closes at random. Why does the mind do this? Is there a way to pinpoint it and leave it open to the present either through medication or surgery?

There is basically a dual or multi existence. The patient is either in the present, past, or some fantasy and to them whichever "reality" they find themselves in currently is the only real world that exists. They cannot distinguish between them. Each one is just as real as the other in their minds. Hallucinations might even be a result of when these "realities" are merging. A fade transition used in a digital slideshow would be an example to give you to explain how they might transition from one "reality" to the other. The difference being this is happening faster than anyone can comprehend.

Long term memory seems to remain intact for the most part. Short term memory is eroded and distorted. Especially in some of the earlier stages it seems a patient can tell you in vivid detail of an event from 30 years ago yet cannot tell you what they just ate for breakfast or if they even had breakfast. In some ways, short term memory or the retarding of it seems to be a possible trigger to this "doorway" of the mind we discussed earlier. I have too little knowledge of this disease and results of dementia results to explain this thought in greater detail. The best advice I can give on this is when the episodes occur handle them as if they are the only true reality at this moment. The patient is living in that partly moment of time in their mind. If they think you are their parent, then play along with them. It can be unsettling and frustrating to you, however they cannot tell the difference. Do not attempt to correct them nor alter the scene playing out before them. An attempt at correction could result in frustration, confusion, and an outburst of anger from the one with the disease. It is better for everyone involved to just go with it.

The patient and the care giver are both doing battle with this disease. The biggest difference is the caregiver survives the war. We might be a little battle worn and suffer a few scars, but we do survive. The same cannot be said of the patient. Everything we encounter in our lives are steps along a journey. We learn from each thing we experience in life. It is up to us just what we learn from these and what we do with that knowledge.

Life is never quite the same after having been in the role of caregiver. I still have a recurring dream that my mother is still alive. Instead of being thrilled and I am terrified. I feel the presence of evil and know this incarnation of her is here to harm me. My mind begins to spin out of control, wondering how she could be alive. It cannot really be her. How did she snap back to normal? Then it hits me she will reverse back to the disease and still die anyway. I then go onto wonder how she is alive and normal with no lasting effects from the disease. Finally, I ask does she remember going through this ordeal? It's needless to say, that when I awake from this dream each time it is not a pleasant experience. I can only guess there are so many unanswered questions along with damage from stress that my mind seems to be making an attempt to resolve these issues.

My image of a caregiver is like the hero at the end of an action suspense thriller that makes it out alive against extreme odds. He walks slowly looking at all the damage left around him. Everyone tries to make him into a hero and keeps congratulating his efforts. He doesn't feel much like a hero, no one was saved, the one he was protecting died anyway. He failed his mission. So, what was really accomplished? All he wants now is to keep walking and to be left alone. He has his own demons to exorcise now and will have to answer for himself if he did all he could. A hero? No. A survivor? Maybe. Only time will tell.

Chapter Thirteen

MOVING ON: LESSONS FROM LIFE

My parents may not have been perfect, but they were the perfect parents for me. I look back on who they were and how and what they taught me. My parents were old school; they taught more by example than by word. They lived their lives in such a way that we knew what was right and what was wrong. They didn't have to punish their kids because we knew they meant business. We, in turn, had a respect for their authority. Being a male, I naturally had a few times when I tested those boundaries and always knew when I was getting too close.

As I stated earlier, I never wanted to do anything that would cause harm to my parents in anyway. I can recall a time when my father asked me about my activities one particular night and why I didn't call to let them know I would be so late. I was very surprised he was not mad he was hurt. He had been very worried about me, and I could see the disappointment in his eyes. That hurt me more than any physical punishment might have ever inflicted. The thought of letting him down was enough to make sure that never happened again.

Have you ever stopped to consider how many times this scene has played out between us and God? If we could see His Eyes or His face when we mess up or sin, I wonder if that would stay with us and haunt us each time we were tempted. I could not even begin to imagine how many times God has been hurt over me doing something really stupid. I can almost see Him in the character of Uncle Jed (from *The Beverly Hillbillies*) as he looks at Jethro and shakes his head, saying that one day he is going to have a long talk with that boy.

Yes, mistakes are a huge part of life. We all make them—some of us more than others. The trick is how we react to or learn from these mistakes. Anyone can screw up, that is only human; however, not everyone can learn from these times. If you are a Christ follower, how you recover from these mistakes can have a huge influence on those who witness your reaction. It's much easier to admit your failure and just pick up the pieces and move on. If we tend to keep trying to cover up mistakes or failure, then when we finally are forced to deal with it, we have a much bigger mess on our hands.

My parents were not always perfect, nor did they always have the right answers. I do know they loved me and did everything they could to make sure I had a better quality of life than they had. Their goal was for things to be easier for their children. Ironically, many of the values they taught and passed onto us were not things they intentionally tried to teach us. They just lived their lives before us, and we learned from watching them. It does not matter who you are; there is always someone watching you, and whether you realize it or not, you are teaching someone something positive or negative.

I understand that many things in our DNA are set in stone and can't be changed, and other things can be. My goal in life has been to take the characteristics that were positive in both my parents' lives and focus on developing them in my life. I did not inherit every single attribute, so I can only strengthen the ones that are present in my wiring. I also realize bad characteristics are there as well, so I try to acknowledge what those are and make sure I work on changing those from bad to good. This is not something I can do on my own, and I trust God to help me develop these into what they should be. Perfection is not my goal. I know that could not be achieved this side of heaven. My goal is to make the most of what I have been given in life.

  We are given no choice in who we are born to, when we are born, or when we die. We are, however, given absolute control over the choices in everything we do with the time spent in between. Having experienced the loss of so many close to me, including my parents, it makes me appreciate just how short and unpredictable life is. If I learned nothing else from all these tragedies, it is the fact that I need to make the most of the time I have on this earth. Anything we gain will not matter a thousand years after we have gone. The legacy we leave through those that we have been in contact with, will still live on.

  I am in no way trying to imply I am perfect or have all the answers. I am just like you I have questions and seek the answers. I fail, get angry, and sometimes hurt others. We all are the same in this way. I am just saying that I have tried to learn from those who have gone before me. It's like when an older person says I wish I had listened when older people told me they wish they had listened to the older people that told them they wished they had listened. Get the point? Wisdom many times comes with age, and although it might be too late for someone to make corrections in their own life, maybe they can pass that wisdom onto a younger person and help them to avoid the same mistake.

We have no guarantee of tomorrow, so living each day as if it is your last is not a bad idea. The fact is, one day it will be your last. I've also wondered if we knew when we were going to die, where would we be when that appointed hour appeared?

I think that it would only make sense if we live our lives as if every day is our last, that we would spend our time doing things that would have a positive impact on people and the world. My personal motto has always been to leave this world a better place than when I entered it. I have never accomplished anything that has changed the entire world; however, if I can make a difference in just one life, then I am one step closer to that goal. Remember, you never know what a kind word, helping hand, or just a smile will do to change a person's day or even their life.

Compassion for others is something that seems to be less obvious today. When a major disaster strikes, we see people ready to help, yet before then, did they ever even give a second thought to the same people? Why is it we must wait for bad things to happen in order to do something good? Jesus tells us that no matter what we do for the least of these, we do for Him. In other words, the small things matter as much as the big. Think about this: What harm would it do if each of us did something nice each day for just one person we encountered? It might even make this a better place to live.

In July 1984, I went on a mission trip to West Virginia. The youth of my church went to help a new church build their congregation through teaching backyard Bible clubs to children in the community. This planted the seeds for missions in my heart. I would not see this until many years later. That trip, along with the life and death of my parents, opened an entirely new direction in my life. I suddenly realized after I got to Brentwood Baptist Church how missions were an avenue to use to work on my kingdom-building goals of leaving this world a better place. We can talk all we want about how we wish the world was better; however, until we take action to change it, it's just talk. The missions minister at Brentwood, Scott Harris, has taught me many things in this area over the years. Kim Cox, the assistant missions minister, has also been extremely helpful in helping me see the world more through God's eyes than through my own. I have traveled to many countries in this world and have seen many types of people.

The one area I have been most troubled by is how it always seems other people groups have so much more faith and desire to worship than Americans. We are supposed to be a Christian nation, and it seems we are farther from it than many developing nations. This is especially true in areas where there are no formal churches and people meet in houses for church and sometimes underground home churches. No matter if it's the United States, Europe, Asia, South Africa, or Southeast

Asia, I have found there is no shortage of hurting people. There are always people seeking a better way or just looking for hope.

One person I met I will never forget. A few years back, I was with a group visiting home churches in a rural area in India. It seemed everywhere we went people thought we could pray for them and heal anything that was wrong with them. They assumed that since we looked different from them and were from America, we somehow had a better relationship with God. This really bothered me because it seemed so obvious their faith was much stronger.

On that trip, a young lady came to us with her young son who had been blind from a very young age. The desperation and pleading in her eyes completely bored straight through my heart. The only thing this mother wanted was for her son to see again. We would later learn that she had TB, and instead of getting treatment, she was spending all she had on her son. She had no desire to help herself until her son was healed.

We did pray over her son, and we made sure she understood not all healing was instant and God didn't always choose to heal everyone. We did connect her with an eye specialist and helped her get her son to one of the top hospitals. I'm not sure what the outcome is on this situation, but the last word was that there was some hope, and that there might be a procedure to correct his eyesight. My point in telling this story is to show how unselfish the mother was in her pursuit, ignoring her own serious health issues to seek help for her son. Something that still bothers me is how little faith we had. We were already discounting God would give the little boy complete healing without a doctor. We were using our Western minds, which are just not used to seeing God move in powerful ways. We had made sure to tell the mom that not all healing was instant. If we had displayed more faith would the little guy have been able to see? Did we doubt God could heal or just thought He wouldn't? Why did we think this way? All this lady wanted was for her son to be able to see! Perhaps we missed out on a huge miracle due to small faith or maybe healing was denied because they would have worshipped us instead of God. We'll never know. Several years have passed, yet I still see those eyes in my mind. When someone seems to completely have no hope and is desperate for any solution, there is no way that ever leaves your memory.

I was finally able to understand that although my mother had never traveled to another country or participated in any official mission trip, she was in fact making any place she happened to be, a mission field. She had no idea that was what she was doing. She didn't wake up one morning and think, *you know I don't have the money to travel, so I'll just show God to those around me through my life*. She just lived her life as who she was, and God did the rest. There is no need for special skills, training, and travel or to even be a so-called missionary to make a difference. The secret is quite simple and might shock you. The key is, just to be yourself and let others see God in you through your actions. If they ask why you act a certain way or why you do a certain thing, you can simply just respond by giving the answers to three short statements: this is who I was;

this is how God changed me; and this is where I am now. Why do we always seem to overcomplicate things?

Many times, in my life, I have wondered if I was born in the wrong era. Something inside of me longs for a simpler time, a more idealistic time when family and morals were more important than the pursuit of money and material things. I think back to how one set of grandparents were textile mill workers, and the other set were sharecroppers. I noticed a few things they each had in common: they lived simple lives, worked hard, and valued family. They worked hard to survive and feed their families, not to buy useless things to impress their friends and neighbors. They bought what they needed. I think it is sad that so many have lost that work ethic. Too many people today think that the world or the government owes them something. People seem to be so self-absorbed that the only thing that matters to them is what they can get out of life.

This reminds me of a question: Do you know your neighbors? Do you know their names? Have you ever spoken to them, other than to say hello? Do you just give them a wave? I hear people talk about the time when neighbors used to look out for one another and help each other. They wonder why that is not the way it is anymore. Why would you expect someone to offer to help you when you hide from them? Maybe a first step to getting back to that type of environment is as simple as introducing yourself to your neighbor. What can it hurt? You might actually meet your new best friend.

It seems each day I am more and more glad my parents were not money centered. This may have been influenced by the fact they never had any money. My parents grew up poor and were not wealthy during their adult lives. They did know what was important in life. God, family, and friends, mattered. I am very thankful for them having raised me this way. After I came to the same conclusion about money, life was much better. I would not trade the true love of family and friends for any amount of money in the world. The money might seem nice at first, yet what kind of meaningful interaction can you have with money? Oh, you will have plenty of "friends" hanging around, but once that money is gone, let's see how long they stay. No sir, don't give me the desire for money. Give me a loving family and true friends any day of the week.

I had a great reminder of this when I went to the Philippines to visit the family of my then current girlfriend. We were on Camotes Island, and the only mode of transportation is motorbike. We were riding through the countryside, and I observed the structures that people were calling home. I also noticed how much poverty seemed to exist. I saw fishermen and farmers, and all were hard at work supporting their families. I was fighting back tears thinking of how blessed I have been and how much I take for granted. Then something struck me almost everyone was smiling. How could these people actually be happy? They didn't have expensive cars or designer clothes. Why were they happy? I had to wonder if the reason was simply the fact they had not yet been corrupted by the lust of money. I enjoy a capitalistic republic such as America and thank God for the opportunity to be able to pursue whatever dreams I have; however, many people get caught up in the money trap and become obsessed with it. They see that a little felt good, but a lot was not enough.

Going to these island villages was almost like stepping back in time. A time where things didn't revolve around working to buy the latest tech gadget that had hit the market or the newest video game system. I know they longed for an easier and better life, yet they seemed content with what they had. I couldn't help to think that they have it made, and I truly pray they and their beautiful paradise are not ruined by progress. I hope they will be able to make a better life for their families, yet not at the cost of destroying what they currently have. Other areas such as Manila and Cebu have given into the influences of the West. Some have really helped their country; however, others have allowed the bad in as well.

I was grateful for this experience. It's nice to be reminded of the simple things of life. I realize we all must work in order to survive, yet our idea of survival is somewhat distorted at times. Some things are just a part of advancing a civilization, but we must also hold onto the important concepts as well, such as family and morals.

Many times, we will read an article on the Internet or in the paper that will say something about backward southerners or outdated views of rural areas. Most of the time they are talking about someone who still holds firm to the Word of God as being truth. In today's culture, that is looked at as a negative thing for some reason. We tend to forget it is God who made this nation what it is, and the more we try to push Him out of it, the more likely it is He just might grant our request. I hope and pray that day never comes.

I was born in the South and have lived my life there. My parents were from rural areas and didn't have the money or luxury of getting college educations. My father actually dropped out of school at an early age to go to work to help his family. The truth is they were not dumb hicks. My father could keep a running balance of his checkbook in his head. He had a knack for numbers and math. I know some people with several degrees who can't even balance a checkbook.

I am proud of my parents and where I am from. We should never be ashamed of who we are or where we are from. Those are the very things that have shaped and molded us into who and what we are now. Unfortunately, we tend to listen too much to Hollywood telling us who we should be, how to look, and how to dress. We need to learn to stay true to ourselves.

We need to also realize that no one is better than we are, nor are we better than anyone else. That is what being created equal is about. Just because one person had more opportunities than someone else or caught a few more breaks doesn't make them any better. We should be happy, not jealous, when others succeed, and we should strive to reach success ourselves.

One last thing I have learned in life is that you must know what you believe and why you believe it. When it is necessary, stand for what you believe in and stand firm in that belief. Don't let anyone tell you what you think or what you believe. Think for yourself!

I have often thought that when my funeral is preached, the main take away won't be how much success or fame I had in this life. I would rather have people leave, talking about how I cared more for others than myself, I was very generous, and that I made a difference! Am I at that point yet? No, I am not there yet. I'm also still breathing, so there is still time for me to live my life in that manner. How we lived is more how we will be remembered than how much was in our bank account or how big our flat-screen was. What legacy are you leaving?

Chapter Fourteen

~

LESSONS FROM DEATH

Death. No one really talks about it or wants to talk about it. We seem to have this idea that if we don't mention anything about it, then perhaps it will overlook us. Good try ...except that it's not going to happen. If you were born, you will face death. The only guarantee in life is death.

What is it we are afraid of? Are we afraid of the unknown? No matter what our reason, no one truly wants to die. A person may say he or she is prepared for death, but I don't know of anyone who hopes they will die anytime soon. When was the last time you met someone who stated they were hoping today would be their last day on earth? As a living, breathing creature, we have an inborn instinct of self-preservation. We will fight to keep alive.

I had the unique opportunity to see both my parents as they were facing death. The battles they faced were different in some ways and alike in other ways. Unfortunately, no matter how gallant the fight, death will eventually win over each of us. I was able to learn probably as much from my parents through their struggles with death, as they had taught me throughout life.

Some of the things I learned were subtle, others not so subtle. My parents were both bedridden by the time they faced their last days. Death does not always announce its arrival or give us any warning at all. They

both had long settled any doubt of where they would be spending eternity. I could take comfort in the fact that as they were facing a certain death, they faced a certain future as well. They focused on their battles knowing that Jesus was waiting at the finish line.

I think that strength and unselfishness were two of the characteristics I noticed. I never once heard a complaint or a "Why me?" asked. Instead, I saw resolve and determination in facing horrible diseases. It was also apparent there was no fear of death itself. I count it as something very special to have watched as a saint of God passed from this world into the next. The comfort of knowing they were now experiencing the truth of their faith was reassuring.

This led me to ponder the fact that not everyone has this reassurance at death. It is really heartbreaking to think that some people watch their loved ones die and have no idea of what awaits them. Even worse is when they do know what awaits them, and it is not heaven.

It seems so many people want to wait until the last possible second to secure their eternal destination. They may not have that luxury. Many are afraid they will miss out on something or not be able to live life to the fullest if they give their lives to Christ and live for Him. Ironically, it is the opposite that is true. Jesus said He came to give life, and He was giving it to us in order for us to live more abundantly. Did He say He would give us a bunch of rules to follow and a long list of dos and don'ts? No, He offers just the opposite. He wishes to set us free from that type of life.

 This just screams at us to tell everyone we know and meet just exactly what Jesus has to offer. The most important thing is to live our lives in a way that clearly shows Christ living in us. There is no need to hit anyone over the head with a Bible and pound Scripture into them. The Bible says in John, that they will know we are Christians by our love for one another. Also, Paul writes that they will know us by our fruit. In other words, if we live as if Christ were in us, then people will see Him shining through. They will see that there is something different in our lives. They will want to know why we are able to face tragedy and pain so well. They will wonder why we only laugh or smile when others get angry during the same type of situations. I am not going to say Christians are perfect or always respond correctly. We are human, and that will never change. We still make mistakes, and we still get angry or make the wrong decisions. The difference is that we have the Holy Spirit living in us, and this helps in our decision making.

 If we have truly allowed Christ to have control of our lives, then we will strive to be more like Him. This will eliminate much of the behavior that would contradict this lifestyle. However, not everyone is at the same stage of their journey to become more like Christ, and therefore, might be prone to more mistakes. Do not expect someone who says he is a Christ follower to be perfect if so, you will both be let down. Humans are just that, human, and will make mistakes. The difference might be in how those mistakes are handled.

There is an old story that goes something like this. Two men are arguing over whether living a moral life is worth it or not. The one man says he wants to enjoy life and party and live life to the fullest every minute. He wants to enjoy every second, indulging in whatever pleases him. The other man wishes to live a moral life and put others ahead of himself. The conversation turns to the subject of when it's time for them to die and they enter eternity. The first man says, "What if you were wrong, and you missed out on all the worldly fun, and you die and just cease to exist?" The second man replies, "What if I'm right?"

The discussion of what happens to us after we die has gone on since the beginning of time. Sadly, some people live their lives as if it does not matter. They trade seventy or eighty years of selfish pleasure for an eternity in hell. The truth of the matter is that we will all experience eternal life. Yes, I said all of us have eternal life after we die. However, there are only two choices of where we spend that time, and it is either with Christ in heaven or separated from Him in hell.

I know some of you are thinking that is very narrow-minded and not inclusive. I am only relaying what Jesus stated when He said He was the only way to heaven. He said no one comes to the Father except through Him. God would love for everyone to enter heaven; however, not all will choose to do so. He loves us so much that He was willing for His Son to die in our place to allow us the opportunity to enter heaven when we deserved hell instead. The point is, we are all born with a sin nature we want to please ourselves. The punishment for sin is death. We all have sinned and thus fall short of God's standard of holy and perfect, which is required to enter heaven.

This created a problem. It meant that no one would be able to go to heaven. God decided His love for us was so deep and He longed enough for our fellowship that He allowed His Son to leave heaven and live on the earth as a human. Jesus was all man and all God on earth and lived a sinless life and died on a cross for us. He took our sins upon Himself and bore the punishment that was rightfully ours. Did you catch that? We are sinful, and He was sinless, yet He chose to take the punishment that was meant for us! The story doesn't end there. He died and was buried then resurrected Himself after three days. That simply means He defeated death. Now death no longer holds us captive. By His sacrifice and defeat over death, we are now eligible to live forever with Him in the presence of God!

It amazes me when I stop to think about how much God loves me. The question always comes up, as to Why? What did I ever do to deserve His love? The answer might surprise you nothing. In fact, as a sinful human I have done more to deserve death and hell than to earn the love of God. That is exactly the point; we could not earn God's love!! He freely gives it. He clearly states in His Word, the Bible, that anyone is eligible for His forgiveness. That really humbles me at times, when I think of some of the really stupid things I have done. It honestly blows my mind that He can love me enough that I would be forgiven.

I have been to ten countries some multiple times as a missionary over the past fifteen years, and the one question that people always have about God is, how do you earn salvation? There is absolutely nothing you can do to earn God's grace. The very definition of grace is "an unmerited favor." Simply put, God loves us and offers salvation to us for free. Every religion I have encountered in various parts of the world has rules to follow and work that must be performed in order to hopefully please their god or gods enough to gain favor. A true follower of Christ will not work to get into heaven; he will do so-called good works as a result of having Christ living in his heart.

I hope no one takes this message wrong. A life lived for Christ is not automatically an easy life. There is no magic formula that will suddenly take away all your debt, give you plenty of money, cure all your sickness, etc. In fact, in some countries people are actually killed for accepting Jesus. Others are persecuted for their belief in Him. One thing Jesus does promise us is that He will never leave us or forsake us. He has already faced the same difficulties and temptation that we have faced, and He knows what that is like to endure. He will go with us through everything we face. He never said He would get us around or out of what we are facing. He said He would go through it with us. Did you see it? "Through it" means we will still have times of heartache, pain, and sickness, along with the happy times. The difference is He will be there with us. Sometimes we are asked to endure these hardships in order that someone else might see Christ through us. Sometimes, it maybe to just simply know what others are going through and thus be able to help them.

Death can come at any time, or a disease or accident can rob us of mobility or our minds. We never know how long we have on this earth. We tend to think that life is measured in years lived. We think we will all grow very old, then we will die peacefully in our sleep. That is just not the case. We never know how long we must live or how long we will have quality of life. I'm just saying that if you think you have plenty of time to decide, you may be wrong.

I have said all this in order to let you know that you have two choices for eternity. It's very simple to know for sure where you will go after you die. My question for you is this: Do you know?

Chapter Fifteen

~

MAKE IT COUNT

The events in this book were not very pleasant to live through and reliving them again has not been much easier. I hope that telling these events and what I've learned from them will in some way have a positive influence on someone. I have felt the need to put this in writing for a long time, and things finally aligned to where it seemed the time was right. If you are still reading, I wish to thank you for your interest and for staying with the story to the end.

If you picked up this book thinking you would read of how to deal with life after the loss of someone you loved, you will be surprised to learn it is too late at that point. The only way to have peace is to make sure your relationship is solid during life. You can't wait until they are gone. You may now ask, what is the key to this? The answer is simple: it's all about relationship.

I can truthfully say I have no regrets about my relationship with my parents. We were able to work through any differences long before they died. I can rest easy in the fact that nothing was left undone. There are too many people who must live with the regrets of things said or left unsaid. If you truly love someone, tell them, and show them now! You may not get another chance.

Do not be afraid to say, "I love you." If a relationship is broken, find a way to fi x it. If the other person will not allow you to repair it, then at least you can know you did your part. Nothing is sadder than someone having to live with regrets of the past. Life has too many problems to add any more to it.

I will offer some rather obvious advice that we so many times fail to follow. Whenever you are with people you love, especially family and friends, play tourist. Take as many photos and videos as you possibly can. Make sure you capture those memories. Save little things such as a handwritten note or a special card. It may seem silly now; however, it could one day become one of your most prized possessions. Do not take for granted that there will be time later for such things. There are no guarantees.

Take a little extra time to spend with those special people. I really don't think an extra five minutes spent chatting or making a phone call will throw off your busy schedule. If you can't make time for family and friends, you may wish to rethink your schedule and your priorities.

Ask yourself two very important questions: How am I spending my time? What matters most to me? The answer to these just might surprise you. If you see you are putting too much time into your career or hobbies, then ask yourself, why? Think about which is really more important to you.

These are not the perfect solutions to enduring the heartaches and pain of life. This is only a list of a few suggestions that do make it easier to cope. Your pain will not magically go away, and you will not automatically breeze through the grieving. I can promise you that it will make it much easier to endure.

So, you've had solid relationships, and you've savored all the memories; yet when that special person in your life dies, you still have a rough time. What now? That is a very good question. A question, in fact, probably asked by everyone who faces such a situation. I wish I had the perfect answer, but I do not. I can only share with you my experience and how I made it through. I hope something somewhere in the pages of this book have been helpful in doing that. That has been the purpose in writing it.

From a very young age, I have faced the death of a loved one many times in my life. I am not able to remember a time in my life where there was not the loss of someone close to me. It's difficult, and it does not get any easier each time. I've been very fortunate to have God in my life and wonderful friends who have been there for me. When someone is grieving, we seem to think we need to say the right thing to them. The truth is, sometimes saying nothing at all is best. A knowing smile or hug can be just the perfect thing. Maybe it just takes being quiet and listening to the grieving person share about how they feel.

Instead of offering "if there is anything I can do for you" statements, just go ahead and actually do something. The needs are obvious during times of grieving, and many times it can be as simple as just being a friend who listens or someone who takes care of the little details.

Death is never a pleasant experience. No one wants to lose a loved one, especially if they seem to die before their time. We have questions, and we have anger and fear. Each person grieves differently, and it takes longer for some to recover than others. I would never pretend I can give you a five-step plan to making grieving easy. My best advice is to actually grieve. You are hurting, and you feel lost go ahead and cry. Take some time away from work and everyone and just get away.

One of the best things to do is talk about the one you have lost. Don't hide your feelings or lock away your memories. Use those wonderful memories as a way to always keep that person with you. This is where the photos and videos you have made will come in handy. Go ahead and wear out those photos from looking at them over and over. Keep their memory alive in your heart. Be careful not to get stuck in the past, though. Life still goes on, so you must also.

The anniversary of a death can be really difficult, especially if it is on or near a major holiday. Take the time to remember those good times and use this as a day of reflection on how you were touched by this person or to remember why they were so special to you.

I realize that just after you lose someone close to you, there will be days when you feel anxiety, loss, anger, and deep pain. You will hate the world and be very bitter. There is no magical solution to avoid this; it's a natural part of grieving. I would suggest that you make sure you have a phone number of a close friend who will allow you to vent. A true friend will do this for you. If you are the friend, be patient and listen to what is really bothering them, and then if you must speak, you'll know better what to say.

It takes time to deal with these feelings. Remember that you must deal with them. Alcohol and drugs are not the way to cope. These only temporarily numb you and can lead to even worse problems. If your friends offer to help you, then allow them to do that. If you have a friend going through a similar experience that you have endured, then by all means share with them how you made it through. Many times, just knowing that someone else has shared the same feelings or experience is very valuable. You both might even get help from your time of sharing.

We go through things in life for a reason. I honestly feel that many of the tough times and tragedies are to not only help prepare us to face tougher things, but also to allow us to be able to help others. Everyone learns something from each experience in life. If you've had to endure something painful and you know anyone going through something similar, please help them through it.

I can only offer advice from the standpoint of being a Christ-follower. It might sound like a cliché; however, He will be there for you. There might be days when it feels you are a million miles away from God, but He has not left. You may be asking, if this God is so great and loves so much then why does He allow all the suffering? I can only say I do not know why He allows these things. You must remember His original intent was to create us for fellowship with Him. He created a perfect world and only asked man to not do one thing, and man failed at that.

That disobedience opened the door for sin to enter the world. As a result, death was part of the consequences. It will always be a part of this world; however, we are promised a day when there will be no more sorrow and no more pain.

I know my loved ones who have died are enjoying that promise. I also know that I have made sure I will also, and as a result, we will be reunited again in the future. Maybe then we will know why some of the things had to happen.

My question for you would be, do you know? Are you sure of your eternal destination? If you answer no, or "I don't know," then please take a few minutes to find a friend or pastor you trust who can explain to you how to know for sure. We are only given one shot at life, so make it count.

Chapter Sixteen

~

LIFE AND DEATH COLLIDE

Throughout my life, I have had several opportunities to face death. I can relate to how it feels to face the possibility that life may be coming to an end. I sometimes feel like a cat, having nine lives. I have learned things about myself and about life through these events. I mostly have realized that strength and character can be built during the darkest portions of our lives. I include a few of these in this chapter because they affected others as well as me.

As a toddler, I was rather adventurous and loved to explore most everything. My mother had gone back to work, and my Grandmother Sigmon would keep me during the day. She was a shift worker in a textile manufacturing plant and had days free to watch me as my mother worked her first-shift job.

One day I was able to sneak away from the watchful eye of adults, just as any conspiring two-or three-year-old is able to do. I quickly found my treasure chest under the sink of the kitchen cabinet. It was a goldmine for a curious, naive little guy. The story goes that among the various "treasures" was a container of household cleaner that was sealed with a lid that had several holes punched into it in order to allow it to breathe. I'm not really sure what the cleaning solution was, but when it was spilled onto about three-fourths of my body, it had a very harsh reaction with my tender skin. It immediately burned my skin and resulted in a near-panic of my grandparents, parents, and other family.

Fortunately, although painful and slow in healing, it was not life-threatening or life-altering. I am told I spent many weeks wrapped in gauze to protect the tender skin areas that had been compromised by the chemicals. The recollections I have of the incident were flashbacks as a child from being forced under water to rinse the chemicals off my body. Although I thoroughly enjoy being in and around water, I sometimes still have panic attacks when my head goes under water due to this early trauma. I only have slight scars on my thighs that look like faint stretch marks and one other small scar that is barely noticeable. I'm really surprised that after this incident, my mother allowed me to be placed in a daycare for a year or two when my grandmother went back to working days.

I contracted a very severe case of the stomach fl u when I was about four or five years old. I became dehydrated quickly and was so sick that I was placed in the hospital for a week or two. I could not even begin to comprehend what must have been going through my mother's mind at this point. Less than ten years after her firstborn died of the exact same thing, she was going through it again with another son. I would imagine she had to be thinking that it was some kind of cruel joke that God was playing on her. Give her a son, then he dies. A few years later she has another son, and then when he is a preschooler, he suffers the same exact illness that took the life of her first son.

I actually have memories of that hospital stay, and they are not pleasant to me. I can still recall how much agony I was in, and the thought of food made me deathly ill. I was hooked up to IVs for nourishment, and I remember having to face the wall because a very bright light was on the other side of the bed, and it hurt my eyes. I remember that there were always people there. Either my mother or my Aunt Essie was there constantly.

I honestly do not know how my mother endured this. The memory of having lost Steve to a similar situation had to still be fresh in her mind. I actually feel sorry for the doctors, because I am certain she would have made sure everything possible was done to save her baby. If I had died during this illness, I am sure there is no way my mother would have survived with her sanity. Losing one child is horrific; losing two is just unthinkable. I was a very sick little child, and my aunt told me years later that she was sure I was going to die. She could not even begin to think how anyone was going to be able to console Ollie after losing another son. Obviously, I made it through, or you would not be reading this story now. No matter what the reason for my survival, the fact is I survived, and in hindsight many things about that now make sense.

In March 1981, I came down with what I call the Reagan flu. I gave it this name because I was home sick from school on the day President Ronald Reagan was shot. That is the same day that a memory of my mother is forever etched into my memory. I was very weak and dehydrated from not eating and throwing up so much that I was to the point of dry heaves. I went to the bathroom thinking I needed to throw up, and my weakness caused me to kneel as I awaited the inevitable. My stomach was empty, so it was a futile trip, and I was just so weak I had to rest on the floor before making the return to my bed. I had left the door partially opened, and my mother walked by to see if I was all right. The look on her face was one of sheer terror.

A few moments later, I overheard her on the phone with our doctor. I could tell she was not happy with whatever she was being told, and I heard her say she would take me to the hospital herself. A short time later, I heard the doctor talking to my mother, and then he was in my room. He ruled out that I needed a hospital visit, and he gave me a few shots and ordered a steady diet of Gatorade and any type of food that she could get into me.

After I had recovered from this severe bout with the fl u, I was able to learn what had upset my mother so much. She told me that when she saw me on the floor, I was in the identical position that my brother, Steve, had been in just before they took him to the hospital when he died. She admitted it was almost too much for her to handle. Seeing me like that was an immediate flashback to when she had seen Steve. There was no way she was going to let that scene end in the same way. If I had not been able to hold any food in my stomach by that evening, she was determined to get me to the hospital, even if she had to carry me to the car herself.

If I had any idea that seeing me in such a weak condition would have caused such a traumatic flashback, I would have made sure there was no way she could see me kneeling on the floor. I cannot even begin to imagine what that did to her. I recovered fully, and as far as I know, this left no lasting impact on her.

From late winter through early spring of 1986, I went to the doctor to check out a knot that had formed on my throat. It appeared as if I had two Adam's apples. I was having discomfort when I would put on a necktie for work. The doctor sent me to a surgeon to have it tested. He withdrew fluid and told me that if it did not return, there was nothing to worry about; if it did return in a few days, I would have to make another appointment and then schedule surgery because there would be a very strong chance that it was a malignant tumor. The area was as big or bigger the following day. The nodule they had found now seemed very likely to be cancer. Blood tests were performed, and questions asked to determine how my thyroid was functioning. It was performing much too well to the point that it was overworking.

I had a few weeks to think about what was invading my body as I waited for the April surgery date. The surgeon had told me they would be removing at least a portion of my lower lobe in order to get the growth off my thyroid. After a postoperative biopsy and blood test, they would discuss any other needed treatment or medications. I remembered the surgeon using the phrase, "Chances are very likely this is malignant." He did not say it was malignant. I never really allowed the thought of cancer being present to be a reality. I had a peace that it was benign.

I knew my parents were very worried over my surgery. I just did not feel the same sense of doom that they were facing. I discussed it with a girl I had been talking to and trying to set up a date with. I told her that we would have to wait until after the surgery, and she was actually dealing with tonsillitis, so we would not be able to go out anyway. I also talked with a few coworkers, and one had actually had a similar surgery and showed me that the scar heals nicely.

Strangely, I was not bothered by the fact that the surgery might prove I had a tumor or thyroid cancer or that I might not even make it out of surgery. Anytime a person is put to sleep, there is a possibility they will not wake. I knew that the very worst thing that could happen would be to die. Although I was twenty years old, I was at peace with that. How could a twenty-year-old feel at ease about this? The answer is quite simple. In my mind, I knew there were two things on my side. The first was that if God could create me, then He could heal me or use the surgeons to correct whatever the problem was. As long as He wanted to do that, He could. The second was that if this led to my death, then I would be fi ne because I knew I had given my life to Jesus and that He was real, and I would just be going to see Him much sooner than I had ever thought.

There was such a calm and peace about the entire situation that I was actually beginning to look at it as an adventure. The day of my surgery, our pastor, Andy Raines, came to the hospital to pray with me and the family before my surgery. Later he would say that he could tell I was doing fine it was my mother he was more worried about. After we prayed, the nurse came in to give me the shot that is given prior to surgery to make you forget any and all worries. If you have ever had surgery, then you know the one I am talking about. As the medicine was beginning to work its magic, my friend Melissa called my room to talk with me before my surgery. I remember telling her the phone was spinning around on the wall in front of me. I vaguely remember thinking that as the call ended, she realized I was too drugged to carry on a normal conversation.

I was rolled down the hall, then put to sleep. The next thing I remember is thinking *I am awake, so guess I didn't die on the table.* The recovery nurse began telling me to open my eyes, that I needed to wake up. I opened my right eye, then she told me to open the other eye, so I closed that eye and opened the other. She shook her head and told me to now try opening both at the same time. She laughed and said, "Yeah, you are going to be fine." As soon as she turned, I closed my eyes again. All I wanted was to sleep.

After I had left recovery and returned to my room, the nurse came in and gave me a mirror to look at my incision. My neck was about ten times the normal size due to swelling and stitches, but I knew it would eventually go down. The following day, my friends Jimmy and Melissa came to see me. They had told me they would, still I was surprised that they came. That meant so much to me to have friends who were willing to give up a little time to check up on me. I could not talk very loudly yet or eat so well, but I still felt things were going to be ok. A few hours later the doctor entered the room and said he had my results back. His pause seemed like it was hours, yet I am sure it was not even a second. The verdict: the lower lobe had been removed, and the growth had been benign.

The thought in my mind was, *death, you lose; I win.* Although later that night my IV would run out, and blood began to fill the tube. I thought, *okay, maybe I won't be too overzealous in my celebration.* Needless to say, I was happy to know I would have more than the twenty years of life I had already lived. The follow-up test showed that I did not need medication or treatment of any sort. That part surprised me; I had been completely healed.

A few years later in 1988, I was working a job as a quality control lab technician in a chemical plant. I became very ill a few months into the job. After countless trips to the doctor and many weeks of missing work, they could not locate a cause of my illness. I even was given antidepressant medication since many of my symptoms seemed related to either depression or stress. The withdrawal from that medication was as bad or worse than the symptoms that I was already having to endure. This illness took a major mental and emotional toll on me. As rapidly as it had appeared, it began to go away. Then I would become sick again. I soon began to feel it was hopeless to even think I would be able to return to normal health.

I learned a few lessons during this time. I knew I could not do anything much more active than read, so I decided to grab my Bible and read through the book of Job. I soon realized I was nowhere near the helpless and hopeless state he had been in. Somehow, I knew that I had to reach down deep inside and pull myself out of this. I knew that I could not do that on my own and learned that sometimes we must reach the bottom in order to realize that our only hope is in God. I had also decided that even though I was only getting partial pay from one of the two jobs I was working, I would continue to tithe and have faith that God would honor that and allow me to continue to meet my financial obligations.

After a few more weeks, I regained my health and my strength. I was never able to find a doctor who could pinpoint the cause of this strange illness. It basically left me as quickly as it had afflicted me. Possibly some chemical I was exposed to had poisoned my system. I have no idea. I worked there for a few more months, and the illness never returned.

A few more incidents occurred as I was writing this book. About three weeks ago, I woke up at midnight and realized I was not breathing. It was as if something was wrapped around my throat. I tried to cough and finally began to wheeze as I inhaled to cough, although nothing was exhaling. I continued to force myself to attempt to cough. I knew I was getting at least a little oxygen in order to be able to make that faint sound. I then forced out the words "help me." I knew if I could speak, I was breathing again. After what seemed like forever, I was able to cough and eventually clear my throat. I had a cold the next day, so I guess fluid had entered my throat during my sleep and blocked my airway. This was not a good feeling. I never panicked, but I will say I was somewhat unsettled by this. Many different thoughts went through my mind. I realized I was in no hurry to die. My main concern had been to breathe. It did make me stop to wonder what would have happened if that had actually caused my death.

Almost two weeks after this had occurred, I encountered a workday that was extremely windy that entire winter and spring had been very wet and windy. I was walking my route and began to cross the street. I saw one of my coworkers driving down the street, so I knew he either needed to give me something or inform me of something. I continued to cross the street, knowing that he was going to stop in order to give me whatever he needed to hand off to me. As I reached the center of the road, I heard a loud crack and instantly knew a tree had snapped. I realized it was falling toward the spot I had been standing in only a few seconds before. I picked up my pace after thinking it might scatter debris when it hit the ground. As I ran to the other side of the road and up a few houses, the huge oak snapped several power lines and sent them whipping about fifty feet. My coworker told me sparks were flying from the power lines as I ran. He was basically frozen where he was sitting, not knowing where the power lines were going to land. He could not tell for sure which direction the tree was heading.

I was actually laughing when I went over to talk to him. I'm not really sure why I was laughing; this could have been a very bad situation. Luckily it turned out well. Later I would reflect more on how my timing had been just perfect in order to miss the tree and power lines. I actually was sad no one had captured it on video. I thought that would have been cool seeing sparks flying behind me as I ran.

All these events have made me realize we had no control over if we live or die. There are so many things that can take our lives. The main take-away I have from all the experiences is the fact that we had better be ready when our time comes, because there may be no time to prepare at the moment of death.

I learned very early in life that death comes to everyone and that every person will have to deal with the loss of a loved one as well. The biggest lesson I have learned from losing so many members of my family and friends, and from my own close calls is that we all die at some time of something. I don't let that truth hinder me from enjoying my life. I still do adventurous things and sometimes things that might seem crazy or dangerous such as diving with sharks in South Africa or trekking in the jungles of Southeast Asia. I don't go out seeking death, and I hope to live a very long and productive life.

I'll just say I love my life, and I love living. I set out to find adventure in whatever I encounter. However, I know one day will be my last, and I am going to keep living life until that time comes.

Chapter Seventeen

~

HEAVEN ON EARTH

No one looks forward to death, especially their own. It is important that we not overlook the fact that we all experience death. If we pretend, we will escape death, then we are putting our eternal future in danger. Each of us must be willing to take some time to think about what happens after we die.

It is natural for us to fear unknown things such as death. The problem with this fear is that it can lead to a fear of living. We should not be afraid to live our lives. We each are wired differently in some areas, yet similarly in other areas. One of the ways we are the same is that each of us wants to live. Yes, I know some people end their own lives, yet usually that is due to severe depression, addiction, or mental disorder. The majority of us want to live at all costs; this is a survival instinct that is built into our DNA. This could easily be a result that we are eternity minded and therefore we think in terms of living forever. The fact is, we do live forever, just not in the current bodies and place we are in.

If we attempt to go through life only enduring each day, tiptoeing around any danger or perceived danger, we will be miserable. This is the same as when a football coach goes to a prevent defense and plays not to lose, instead of playing to win. The result is usually the same a defeat instead of a victory. Another example would be a driver who is so afraid of getting into an accident that he or she drives well below the posted speed limit and avoids as much traffic as possible. Eventually the fear of the accident will take away any joy or freedom of driving. The same is true when we fear death to the point that we are only existing instead of living.

I bring all this up to just mention the fact that Jesus said He came to give us an abundant life. He didn't say He only wanted to give us life or an ordinary life. He wanted us to enjoy living. We can enjoy life if we treat it more as an adventure to seek and enjoy rather than something we must endure. Each new day should be anticipated, the same as opening a birthday or Christmas present. Actually, each day truly is a gift, a gift of life. We are not guaranteed to live to a hundred; we are not even promised tomorrow. When we awake, we are accepting the gift of another day of life. The key is what we do with this gift.

Each morning we are faced with a choice: What will we make of this day? Will we forge ahead, excited to tackle any challenge we will face, or will we gloomily trudge through another day of traffic and work? Our attitude is very much a factor in what type of day we will have. I'm not promoting the power of positive thinking, just the fact that we can determine the outcome of each day simply by how we act and react. If we let every little thing get us down, then it will surely be a long, horrible day. If we decide to not let minor setbacks ruin our day, then we have a much better chance of having a really good day.

I mentioned abundant life, and I want to take a minute to think about what that means. It does not mean longer life or that every day will be a great day where everything goes right for us. I feel it means we will have a fuller, more fulfilling experience in our lives. We gain much freedom from the rules and regulations of "religion" by following Christ, thus lifting a burden of dread and fear. The dread and fear of trying to live up to a list of dos and don'ts is removed. This alone is enough to make each day easier to face. I'm not going to sugarcoat things and pretend that a life lived for Christ is going to be easy and there will be no more worries. We live in a fallen world ruled by humans who are greedy and selfish, and that means there will be bad days and really bad days just as well as good days. The fact that we choose to live our lives for Christ will not in any way make us immune to hurt, pain, tragedy, or loss.

We must understand that this life is just a dress rehearsal for our eternal life. We have two choices of where that will be spent: either heaven or hell. We have at the most maybe seventy-five to one hundred years that we will live on this planet, so what is that in comparison to eternity? It is a very short time indeed. This life gives us an opportunity to learn more about the God we serve and allows us to learn to be more like Him.

Much of life is relational, and this is a point of Christianity that most people seem to miss. It is all about relationship. Our relationships with God, ourselves, people we like, and people we don't like all, have an effect on the other relationships. That is the area we usually need the most work in. We were created to live in community. That is one reason God made Eve to give Adam a helper and companionship. In the garden of Eden, Adam and Eve had perfect fellowship with their Creator. The original intent of creation was to allow the creation a chance to fellowship and relate to the Creator. We already know that was spoiled through selfish greed of wanting to be like God, yet that desire for a close relationship was already in our makeup and never left. After the opportunity for relationship was restored through God's redemptive plan of Jesus' life, death, and resurrection, man was once again able to fellowship with God.

  Just as we have the desire to fellowship with God, we also have the desire to form relationships with other humans. We choose mates, best friends, and buddies, along with forming relationships with blood relatives. This is one reason that the prison system has the most persuasive form of punishment solitary confinement. No one wants to be alone. We were made for interaction with other humans, and if that is removed, it is as if a part of us dies.

  Yes, I have a point in bringing all of this into this chapter. Part of living an abundant life is that we try to bring a little bit of heaven to earth. Instead of only longing for paradise after we die, we should strive to make this earth more like heaven. If we as Christ followers would actually model the life of Christ more than just talk about it or dream about eternity, then maybe we could make this a more enjoyable place to live. It might be true that we are only on this planet for a short time, yet why not make it as much like heaven as we can? It's really not that difficult to accomplish.

We have been given the greatest gift possible, and we should demonstrate that love as much as talk about it. A person can tell you how wonderful something is all day, yet if they don't show evidence of that in their life, then who will believe them? In fact, others will question if the person doing the talking actually believes it.

I have talked quite a bit about Jesus and Christ followers in this book. This is written for everyone, not just those who have chosen to follow Christ. We are all on this earth together, and we all must live, work, and play with one another each day. There is no reason we should not all get along. If we don't have the same exact beliefs, then that should in no way affect our friendship. I've written this book from the viewpoint of someone who has lived without and with Christ in their life. I have been better at times of demonstrating the difference He has made in my life than at others.

The truth is I am human, and humans will never be perfect. I can strive to follow the example Jesus set for me through His life as a man, yet I will fall short time and time again. Will I still get angry? Yes, I will. Will I still make stupid mistakes? Yes, you can count on it. I can only try to learn from the mistakes I make and strive to avoid making the same ones in the future. Life is about learning. The two best teachers are experience and mistakes. Both can be great teachers if we allow them to be. We can all look back on younger days and shake our heads and ask ourselves just what were we thinking when we did some of the dumb things in the past. That's all a part of living and growing wiser. We all grow older, and hopefully, we grow wiser with our age.

The story of Jesus giving His life in order for others to live was rather easy for me to relate to. I learned at a very young age that my older brother, Steve, had died before I was born. I was able to piece together that, logically, if he had not died, then I probably would never have been born. When I first heard the story of how Jesus' death allowed me to live, it was a simple comparison for me to make. There were some differences, of course, yet the basic idea made sense to me. I know that given the choice, Steve probably would not have chosen to die so a younger brother could be born a few years later. Steve's death in no way forgave my sins or offered me eternal life. The premise is the same, though a life had to be given in order for another to live. Thankfully, the death and resurrection of Jesus did in fact do these things, and I was able to understand them even as a young child by having a very real analogy to compare it with. It was simple to me, just as if Steve had not died, I could not have been born, I also could not have been reborn without the death of Jesus.

Just as I long to meet my brother face-to-face for the first time, I also long to meet the one who made the ultimate sacrifice for me face-to-face as well. Can you imagine the status updates on social networks from people entering heaven? I can just see some of the tweets as well from those who have been there for many years. Something along the lines of "streets are gold for real" or "chilling with Paul." I could give many more examples, yet you get the point. How exciting to think that not only will we be reunited with loved ones, but we will also meet the great heroes from the Bible and history. Even that will pale in comparison to actually meeting the Creator of everything in the universe. If none of this can excite you, then I doubt anything can!

I have very few regrets in my life, yet there are still times I wish life included do-overs. It does not. The past is unchangeable; it has happened, and there is no way we can undo what is already done. Fortunately, we have the chance to learn from the things in our past and make our future better.

Heaven on earth can be more of a reality by just a few simple acts. A smile or wave toward a stranger will do wonders for the other person and us as well. Stopping to enjoy the song of a bird or to watch kids play will brighten your day. Making friends with the person who is not the most popular member of the group can lead to valuable relationships. Remember that Jesus did not associate with the religious, pious elite of His day; instead, He befriended the misfits and outcasts.

If we would just start looking at people as people and not judging their ethnic background, bank account, body mass, etc., then we would find that none of us are really that different. We all have the basic desire to be loved and accepted.

Chapter Eighteen

~

TRINA

Saturday March 27, 2010, began as a beautiful spring day in Nashville. I was glad to be working on a nice day instead of in the rain that had become the normal weather pattern. I knew this was to be a busy day; after work I would need to race home to change clothes in order to attend my friend's wedding.

About an hour before the end of my day, things suddenly changed. I checked the e-mail on my phone and saw something that totally shocked me. A friend of mine who was a softball teammate and also attended my former Sunday school class had been killed in a motorcycle accident a few hours earlier. My plans changed in just an instant from attending a friend's wedding to attending another friend's wake.

I thought how quickly life can change in just a blink of an eye. I also wondered how my friend Trina began her day. I'm sure she was excited to be off work and able to enjoy a gorgeous spring day riding motorcycles with her friends. The thought never would have entered her mind that this would be the last time she ever rode. One minute you are riding along, and the next you wake up in heaven. I must admit, even though we are the ones who mourn and cry, maybe it should be the other way around. A person who dies as a believer in Christ should cry for the rest of for us who are stuck in this crazy, mixed-up world. They are enjoying paradise as we deal with all the consequences of a fallen world.

No one wants to think about how or when they will leave this world. I think it would be nice, though, if we could go out while doing something we truly love and on a beautiful day. This is exactly how Trina left us.

As I mentioned, instead of attending a wedding, I was now going to a wake. There had been a game night planned; however, with this tragic news it was turned into a memorial gathering. Many people expressed memories, thoughts, and reactions. I think this is wonderful therapy for the grieving process. Sadly, too many times we keep our feelings bottled up inside.

The feelings I had upon first hearing the news were shock, disbelief, and a numb feeling. I didn't know what I felt or how I should feel. I have experienced death many times in my life; however, the unexpected deaths are the ones that seem to be the hardest to deal with. I needed to contact a few people to let them know about the news. I looked back at the message once more just to make sure. So many times, bad news is just so tough to accept that we have to convince ourselves that it is really true.

I mentioned earlier that Trina and I both played on the same softball team. Ironically, there was to be a practice scheduled for the very day she died and the following day. I had decided not to sign up due to the event that was scheduled (which would later become her memorial gathering) and also because of my friend Mark's wedding.

The season began in two weeks, and I had no idea how a manager was supposed to address this to a team or how to pay tribute to our fallen teammate. I'd never lost a player before, and this was something totally foreign to me. I could imagine our first game would be very emotional, and there would be difficulty in concentration on the actual game. At the same time, I felt that getting back on the field would be the very best thing for our team. Our team was very tight knit and had a family type of bond. I was convinced we would be better for this experience not better as in wins or losses, better in how we handled daily life and how we interacted with each other and strangers.

As we gathered Saturday night, a thought occurred to me that the reason I was even writing this book was to retell the fantastic events surrounding the death of my mother and to help people as they grieved. It made me wish this project was finished in order to help the forty or so people gathered that night. At the same time, I thought *maybe this is an opportunity from the Lord to better understand what it is I am actually writing about here*. This would allow me a fresh look at the different ways people express and process grief.

Everything concerning this project has seemed to have God's hand on it. I understand having to wait so many years for this to be written; it has allowed be to become friends with the person who would become my editor and begin writing at just the exact time she is experiencing a crisis that helps her understand the angle of this book. I've met so many people with similar stories and experiences, and I can see that there is a need to share these things. Then with my friend's sudden death, I had more experience with different styles of grieving. No way could I have arranged the events leading up to this project or that have developed during its process.

During the memorial gathering as we shared memories and good times, I couldn't help but notice the difference in what and how people choose to remember a loved one. Some were smiling, others laughed, many cried, some stared blankly, and one or two seemed indifferent. I consider all these normal parts of the grieving process. No two people are alike, and thus the differences in grieving styles. Listening as others shared their memories or favorite times was very interesting. Each person painted a different portion of the total portrait of a person. I heard such things as she had a love for Jesus, a great friend, wonderful smile, sweet personality, caring heart, great competitor, good teammate, unselfish player and person. Although these were very diverse attributes, they all gelled to form the image of the person we knew as our friend.

How will I be remembered? That is a question that more and more enters my mind. We all leave a legacy, and each day we write a new page in the book that will be remembered as our life. Some of those books sit on a shelf and collect dust, some are pristine because we are afraid of damaging the cover of such a precious item, and others are well worn with pages falling out due to continual use. Makes me wonder what my life book will be used for, if at all. I had a friend a few nights ago say he will have thirty to forty more years with his parents, and his kids will have

Grandparents due to the fact that his parents are only in their forties, and he is in his twenties. I immediately thought, *you don't know that. We have no guarantee of tomorrow or even one minute from now. We truly need to live each day as if it is our last.*

I know when someone dies, their Facebook page instantly becomes a memorial site where people go to leave their last thoughts and comments. I went to Trina's page to read her friends' comments when I noticed her final status update. I have often changed mine just in case anything happened, and I was unable to ever change it. Hers said something like "a great weekend is over, now it's back to real life." I instantly thought, *Yeah, your weekend was wonderful, and you have entered into real life.*

Think for just a minute. You have plans to enjoy a beautiful, warm day riding motorcycles with your friends. This is a great weekend in your opinion, then suddenly your life ends. This sounds like a terrible end to an otherwise great day, until you stop to think about what has really just happened. A person who truly loved God was out enjoying His creation and the things she loved to do. The sudden end to this life was not an end at all. Stay with me for just a second. What appears and feels like an end for those of us still here is in reality a transition for the person experiencing it. As Paul stated in the New Testament, to die with Christ is to gain. Simply put, a person who has accepted and trusted Jesus transitions from a life on earth to a life in heaven upon death. If we look at it from this view, then it is not a bad trade at all.

At the time of losing someone you love or someone who is a close friend, it doesn't seem to be a good trade. We miss our friend or family member; we miss seeing them and talking with them. Notice that all of this is our feelings. It's what we are missing or what we are deprived of now. Our attention should be on celebrating the wonderful event that they are now experiencing. I know, we are human, and it is next to impossible to feel or think this way in the face of tragedy. I can almost hear them now as they look down from heaven at us and say, "Stop crying already; I'm having the time of my life. Wish you were here!"

The human mind just doesn't normally process this way through grief, so as we work to that point, we need each other. We need memories; we need a shoulder to lean on, an ear to just listen, or a day just to cry. However, you handle grief, go with it. There is no wrong way or no right way to deal with loss. We are all different and respond differently, so no one will ever write a five-step plan to proper grieving. It's life, and life is sometimes unfair and tough. We handle it with whatever method works best for us. I will say one thing that is true: no matter how we deal with it, having Jesus go through it with us is much easier than going alone.

Chapter Nineteen

~

GOOD NEWS ABOUT DEATH

Death and good news in the same sentence might seem rather strange. It actually is more common than most might realize. Unfortunately, as humans, we seem to not learn until something shocking or tragic first gets our attention. Once our focus has been shifted, then we are in a position where we are ready to learn or benefit from whatever event has jolted us awake.

One example I will share is from Trina's accident that you read about in the previous chapter. The gentleman who was the first to arrive upon the scene of the accident had watched how Trina had lived her life. God was able to use Trina's accident, her funeral, and how her friends and family reacted to make this man realize that he had been hiding and running from God for several years. I have not been able to hear his full story, so I will not speculate on anything. I will just retell the basic story that I know. This just shows that even though we may not know anyone is paying attention or that whatever we are doing is making any difference at all, it just might be the missing piece of the puzzle that ties it all together for someone.

My friend Steve's father has been battling cancer for about two years now, and Steve has always had a burden for his father's salvation. He knew that a person can only come to Christ by the Holy Spirit drawing them and through God's pursuit of us. I know this had bothered him for a while, and then the cancer diagnosis did not help his anxiety over the situation. After about a year of this battle and many ups and downs with his health, Steve's father finally realized that God had spared his life. Even though his health was not at 100 percent yet, he was still alive. He was able to understand that God loved him, and that Jesus had died for him, and he finally gave into the tug on his heart from God.

The thing is, God loves us so much that He will never stop pursuing us. We might turn Him away, yet He doesn't let that stop Him from chasing after us. Unfortunately, sometimes we think we have plenty of time and can live our lives before we decide to allow Christ into our lives, and at that point it is too late. We only have so much time on this earth, and once it's gone, it's gone.

My friend Pamela was going to be the coauthor of this book as I set out to bring these ramblings into some sort of a fl ow that could be read. Shortly after we had discussed working on this project together, her mother was diagnosed with cancer, and most of her free time was spent with her mom in Texas. I had finished writing the basic story and what I felt needed to still be fleshed out, and I sent it to her. We thought maybe with this struggle, she would be able to provide a more personal feel to the story. I realized how much of a toll this was taking on Pam, so I told her I in no way expected her to continue with this project unless she felt the need or desire to share her experiences with her mother's battle in this book as well.

I felt I needed to be patient and allow her time to see how this would turn out. Eventually her mother lost her battle, and Pam told me she could not find ways to express her grief, so I assured her it was okay to no longer worry about working on this project. She needed to spend the time sorting things out on her own, in her own way.

The amazing part is that I knew all along that there was just something missing from the overall book, and the long delay allowed me time to learn and experience some things. I was able to go back and add to some chapters and even create others. I felt also by this time that I was the one the Lord was telling to relay the stories in this book, and that I should not take the easy way out by finding someone to help.

Just recently I heard a story from Pam that really touched me, and I wanted to share it here also. It was posted on Facebook, so it is already public knowledge. She recently went on the first shopping trip since her mother's passing. things went well until the end of the trip when she realized that normally she would call her mom and they would talk about what she bought and saw and other experiences. She was quite bummed

by this and told her husband, Zach, about this when she got home. Zach turned to her and said, "I know I'm not her, but I'll listen if you want to tell me." For the record, men hate shopping! Guys, pay attention to what this man just did. He was willing to listen to his wife talk about her shopping experience and relive it with her, because he knew she could no longer do that with her mom.

Something that is as easy and simple as being willing to listen, if only for a few minutes, can have the biggest of impacts. I remember almost every comment about that post was in praise of a husband having so much love for his wife.

Chapter Twenty

~

SO, WHO *REALLY* CARES?

The question might be asked, who cares? It seems everyone likes to keep to themselves. We all have our own problems, so why would we think anyone would be interested in our hurt or problems? Is there someone who truly understands and really cares? The answer may sound like a worn-out cliché; however, Jesus honestly understands and cares. Let's take just a few minutes to look at why this is a true statement. It may seem impossible for the Son of God to be able to understand anything about the pain we humans suffer.

First and foremost, we must realize that when Jesus came to earth, He did come in human form. Even though Jesus was all man, He was also all God. His deity never ceased. Remember, even though He was God in human form, He still felt the same pain and experienced the same emotions as other humans. The Creator lived with the creation as one of the created.

Jesus had many friends, followers, and also enemies during His life on earth. He had a few very close friends, an inner circle if you will. He also enjoyed friendships with others outside this circle. The Bible tells us that Jesus was so moved and so hurt by the death of His friend Lazarus that He wept. The Son of God actually cried when His friend died. We may not have the power to bring our friends back from the dead; however, we can know that Jesus clearly understands what it is to be separated from a close friend by death.

Several times we are told of Jesus being so moved by a person's faith or by their grieving that He restored life to the deceased. He did not raise everyone from the dead, yet He did demonstrate He had the final say on whether or not someone remained dead or was given life.

We can go one step further with His understanding of death. Jesus died Himself! He not only died, but He also willingly laid down His life as atonement for our sin. Let's take just a moment to think about how Jesus died. He suffered humiliation and punishment at the hands of trained killers. Roman soldiers who carried out executions were professionals at their trade. Jesus was whipped and beaten to within one lash of his life. They knew how to inflict as much pain as possible and do the most damage to a human body and yet allow the person to live. I could not even begin to imagine how painful it would be to be scourged with a leather strap that has pieces of bone, metal, and glass embedded into each strand. Imagine just for a moment that each lash caused all these particles to dig deep into the skin as the leather wraps around the body. Flesh, muscle, and ligaments are forcibly ripped and torn as the whip is retracted, only to be used over and over until the prisoner's mutilated body is no longer even recognizable as a human form.

Jesus does not understand pain and suffering? I think He knows much more than anyone. The beatings were just the beginning. His beard was literally ripped and torn by hand out of His face. Adding to this pain and humiliation, a makeshift crown of long thorns was pressed deep into His scalp. Later, He would carry His own cross up a hill until His body could no longer bear the load. The suffering does not end; it gets much worse.

Reaching the top of the hill, His wrists are then nailed to the crossbeam of the cross, using nails which can best be compared to railroad spikes. Next the cross section is attached to the upright, and His feet are nailed together to the upright. Finally, the entire cross is dropped into a hole. Each labored breath causes the already bruised, ripped, bloody tissue to rub against the rough wood, intensifying the pain.

Crucifixion was reserved for the worst of criminals. It was the most brutal and humiliating form of death the Romans used. Yet here we see an innocent man being put through this torture. As you can guess, Jesus died much sooner that many others due to his extreme torture and lack of sleep and nourishment.

Yes, of course, Jesus understands death. He faced death and then overcame it completely. He not only raised people from the dead during His ministry, but He also resurrected Himself! He dealt death a knockout punch and overcame it once and for all. The resurrection of Jesus from the dead proved His power over death. He went through all this so that even though these earthly bodies will age, eventually die, and decay, it is not the end. He endured all this just to allow us to enjoy eternity with Him.

How do we know that Jesus knows how a death makes us feel? He was moved to tears by the death of His friends, He raised others from the dead after seeing the grief of loved ones, He died Himself, and most importantly He triumphed over death.

What does all this mean? How will this help me when someone I love dies? It may not immediately ease the pain or make things any easier, but we can rest assured that Jesus understands; He wants to comfort us. He may not physically appear to us to accomplish this. It maybe that He will put someone in our lives who will be a friend when we need help to face life's difficult times. God created an entire world out of nothing, so it's easy to think He can arrange for just the right people to enter our life at just the right time.

It is comforting to know that our God not only understands what we are facing but has actually faced it Himself in order to show us that. Instead of the T-shirt, He has the scars to prove it.

Chapter Twenty-One

~

SUFFER WELL

There are always people who ask the question, why does God allow bad things to happen to good people? Many times, there are just no answers to this question. I recently heard a term that just might help us to understand this situation better. I heard someone talk about a person who suffers well. Yes, I know, that seems to scream contradiction. If we allow ourselves to take a closer look at this phrase, just maybe we might begin to piece things together.

It seems throughout the New Testament of the Bible that the greatest things God accomplishes come through suffering, trials, or just hard times. No, God does not make people hurt just for laughs; He has a purpose. Many times, if it was not for these difficult times and circumstances, there would be no opportunity for us to show just how powerful God is.

Let's look at this from a purely secular view. Which do we remember more, the championship game with a predictable outcome or the one with a great come-from-behind finish? I'll give you three examples, and you'll better understand my meaning. If I say miracle on ice, Jimmy V's hug, or music city miracle, almost everyone knows what I am talking about. The Lake Placid Olympics, where the underdog USA hockey team defeated the highly favored Russian team to win the gold medal, is only remembered because it should have never happened. Who could forget Al Michaels screaming, *"Do you believe in miracles? Yeeeeeeeeeeees!"* North Carolina State basketball coach Jimmy V. running across the floor looking for someone to hug after defeating a heavily favored Houston team to win the NCAA Championship is a moment in sports that truly captures an unexpected victory. How about the Tennessee Titans' victory over the Buffalo Bills during the playoff s on the last play of the game to advance to the Super Bowl? We would not remember these or other similar stories if there was not something different, something amazing about the outcome.

Many times, when we pray for a sick person or for a tough situation, we tend to ask for healing or a way out. If God only gave us good things or easy lives, then what would that demonstrate? When we face difficult times or nearly impossible odds, we are being given a platform on which to either proclaim God or to deny our faith in His ability. How we react to circumstances is very important to the view of God we give to others. Our actions and reactions reveal how and what we truly believe. The examples I used from the world of sporting events can help us understand similar victories in life.

The way a person handles fighting for their lives after learning they have a terminal illness can truly affect not only themselves and their family, but many others as well. The easiest response is to just give into the disease and die. We all die sometime and from something, right? This would not be an example of suffering well. An example of how to suffer well is someone who hears this devastating news and attacks it head-on. Yes, they will pray for healing, yet also realize that God heals everyone. Yes, you read that correctly; God does heal everyone. We just might not be expecting the healing He delivers. He will either heal someone by restoring their health or by helping them to escape the pain and disease through death. Just because the outcome is not what we hoped for or expected, in no way lessens the fact that God has answered the prayer and brought healing.

A person who suffers well will bring glory to God through the struggle He will acknowledge that God is indeed in charge no matter what the

outcome. Many times, God can use suffering to bring positive changes that otherwise would never have been possible. If a young man finds out he is dying from a terminal illness and all medical hope has been lost, then he has choices. He can become bitter, depressed, and reclusive, or he can make the most of the time he has left. If he chooses the latter, then he will be a better father, husband, brother, friend, or coworker. It seems we too often take things for granted until they are either gone or threatened to be lost. There is an old saying that asks the simple question, why do we wait until we are dying to actually live?

A person who can face certain death or unbelievable misfortune and still give honor and praise to God not only earns respect, but the attention of an unbelieving world. At the very least, people will wonder how he can still have faith. We will face difficult times and difficult choices in our lives. We will not always be able to choose our circumstances; however, we can almost always choose our response. Our response is what people see and remember much more than the circumstances.

The recent flooding in Tennessee is a great example. After entire communities were destroyed, instead of just waiting around for the government to offer a solution, people took action. Many neighbors and strangers came together to help those who did not fare as well during the two days of 17.5 inches of rain. It didn't matter the color of skin, balance of bank accounts, or gender people helped people. As a result, a state and communities survived an unexpected tragedy. The ironic thing is that because the reaction to a natural disaster was so atypical, there was almost no national news coverage of one of the worst weather events in history. It seems that because there was no rioting, no murders over bottled water, and no looting, the national news just didn't seem to deem it worthy. One would think that with so much bad news being reported, that this would have been a story to breathe a breath of fresh air into their reports, yet they chose to focus on other stories.

If nothing else was shown through this bonding, we saw that there are still people who care about someone other than themselves. Everyone helped in whatever way they could. An interesting thing about the floodwater: it didn't pick and choose its victims. The water destroyed property and possessions of blue-collar workers, musicians, doctors, lawyers, waiters, hotel workers, ministers, rich, and poor.

Disaster can strike anyone at any given time, and usually with little or no warning.

This weather event will be talked about for many years to come. It seems the thing more people are already recalling is not as much the tremendous amount of water and damage, but instead, they are focusing on the recovery. More precisely, they have seen how so many strangers became friends through working together to rebuild what nature had destroyed. It would have been easy to just sit back and hope the government helped get things repaired during the next several years. Fingers would have been pointed and blame placed for misdirected funds or slow or no assistance from the government. What transpired was something completely different. People from all walks of life pitched in and helped each other the way neighbors and Americans used to look after each other. You remember those stories: when someone was down, a neighbor would be there to lend a hand to pull them back up off the ground.

These are just a few examples of what is meant by "suffer well." Hopefully, you have been able to grasp a better understanding. The main point is that people will see our story unfolding. We have a chance to write it anyway we choose, so the choice of how to act and react is completely up to us. This is what they will remember, and for those of us who claim to be Christ-followers, we should suffer well, because of our relationship to the one who is in complete control.

Your book, which is the story of your life, still has blank pages to be filled. Each new day brings another opportunity to impact the world around you and those people who live in it. I have just a few last questions for you to ponder. How does it end? What will your story say about your life? Did you suffer well?

Chapter Twenty-Two

WHAT IF?

It is a given, or at least it is presumed that there is no reversal for the onset of dementia or Alzheimer's. In all reality this is probably true, since no case has yet to be reversed that we know about. What if it could be reversed? Think of the possibilities.

This disease has never been easy to accurately diagnose in the early stages. Improvements in the medical field, education, and awareness have made it easier. Think for a moment what if it was misdiagnosed and was only a disease with symptoms that mimicked Alzheimer's. What if there might have been a cure for what was wrong, yet it was mistreated as Alzheimer's and the window of opportunity was wasted?

A few other things to consider. Is it possible that like in the case of autism, that there is actually a brilliant mind still trapped inside a body that seems to be short circuiting? When taking just a glimpse of the outer body it seems to scream there is no intelligent life here! Yet inside the brain is a very intelligent mind hidden deep within. What if in reality the mind is still doing its job? The kicker being that now it must find a new way to communicate. What we call "normal" process of communication no longer works the same way, so the brain and body compensate by developing a new process of communication. If this is the case we need the key to unlock the new code. There is so much we do not know about the brain or how it functions. Research has shown we only use a very small portion of our brain's capacity. So, is this idea really that unfathomable?

What if we cracked the code? If we found a way to tap into this newly altered or reinvented means of communication think of the possibilities. Research into dementia, autism, Alzheimer's, etc. would take a drastic turn. No longer would we just simply give up or settle for the time we have left. It would not be outside the realm of possibility to glean information from the patient on what they think, how they process, and how life appears to them. So many questions could be answered.

We would need to consider the unintended consequences as well. If this code were cracked, it would possibly just be a temporary reprieve and the patient might once again succumb to the disease. The obvious questions would then be, do we put ourselves through this pain again and more importantly is it fair to subject the patient to the entire degenerative process again? At this point, all this is just hypothetical, yet both the positive and negative must be considered.

If this were to somehow materialize it might only allow for a few additional short months with a dying loved one. Time is precious, who wouldn't want to add a few more weeks or months of quality time with someone they love? Then again, the information collected just might lead to a productive treatment, or maybe an eventual cure not only reverses the disease, but also restores and repairs the damaged areas of the brain. WOW! The possibilities are endless. Research must continue and all ideas explored.

I realize all research seems to point to a degeneration and regression of the brain. The patient's brain begins to forget or unlearn how to do things. Here is my point...what if...

Yes, these are the questions we must keep asking. This is a horrible disease and a brutal enemy. We cannot stop fighting until the war is won!

What if...

Chapter Twenty-Three

~

WELCOME HOME

Ollie looked at her family gathered around her bedside and closed her eyes one final time. As her eyes opened again, she was standing in the most beautiful flower garden she had ever seen. The aroma from the flowers was intoxicating, such soothing and relaxing fragrances. She immediately wondered who owned this lovely garden. She continued to explore the seemingly endless floral.

A tall young man quietly approached her. Slightly surprised, she looked up into a warm, kind face and thought, *oh this must be the gardener*. "Sir," she asked, "are these your beautiful flowers?" He replied with a kind smile and placed His strong hand upon her shoulder, saying, "These actually belong to My Father." He bid her to follow Him, and He would show her around. Ollie followed Him, and soon they were at a beautiful open white gate of excellent craftsmanship. She marveled at how it appeared to strongly resemble a pearl.

Shyly Ollie said, "I'm sorry. I failed to introduce myself." As she was about to tell the kind, handsome stranger her name, He laughed and said, "My child, I already know you. Soon you will understand." She thought, *He does remind me of someone, and it seems I have the feeling we have been friends for years*. Yet still she could not quite place the face.

As if reading her mind, He turned to her and smiled knowingly and said, "Yes, we first met many years ago when you were a mere child. I wanted to greet you personally and show you your reward." "Reward?" she asked. "Did I win some contest?" At this the young man burst into hearty laughter. "No, My child. It was no contest. You were faithful in little, and now you will be rewarded greatly."

Still somewhat confused, she said, "I really don't understand." He simply smiled again and said, "Soon you will see for yourself. We need to walk a little further, then you will meet some people who wish to talk to you. Don't worry; there is plenty of time to see everything and to answer all of your questions. Actually, don't even think about time, because time does not matter here."

The young man stopped beside the purest stream Ollie had ever seen. He pointed to a small rock, and they sat there listening to birds sing and watching butterflies drift gracefully by. He then turned to her and said, "My dear, sweet child. I've looked forward to this day when I would be able to welcome you home. The name you will know Me by is Jesus." At this, she instantly recognized Him. Only now could she see the scars in His hands. Suddenly, tears filled her eyes, and she immediately bowed before her Lord. He gently patted her shoulder, and as she sat up, He softly wiped away her tears. He said, "I wanted to thank you for a job well done." Shaking her head, she mumbled that He must have been mistaken; after all, what had she ever done? He gazed into her eyes and stated that her humility was one of the things He had enjoyed watching most in her life. "I will let you see for yourself what an impact your selfless acts and kind words had upon so many people."

They stood and continued to follow the road that she now realized reflected a light whose source she had not yet located. There appeared to be no sun, yet everything was bathed in a radiant glow. Looking back at the road, she realized it was almost transparent with a hint of a golden hue. Jesus turned to her and said, "Yes, this is pure gold." She asked, "Should we walk on it? I would hate to get it dirty." There was more laughter and a reassuring answer: "Although My Father owns it all, He freely gives it to you to enjoy."

Around the next bend they stop, and he suddenly raises one hand a long line of people appears. Shyly she says, "Oh, I see there are many people waiting to see You." This results in the loudest laugh yet. "No, my child, they are not waiting to see Me. They have been waiting to talk to you." "Why would they wait to talk to me?" she asked, with a confused look. "You see, these are all the people that you in one way or another influenced to accept Me into their lives. You were the one I chose to enter their lives in times and ways that no one else could reach them. It was your life and your faithfulness to Me that allowed them to see Me through you. I'll give you time to talk with a few of them, and you'll understand more completely."

The first in line were two small children. They excitedly ran up and threw their arms around her neck and kissed her cheeks. "We only knew you as the cookie lady from vacation Bible school; we never knew your name.

We enjoyed the classes and the games; although, we didn't understand much about the Jesus they were telling us about. We finally understood after you gave us extra snacks and a hot dog when we told you that what we ate there would be our supper. We were able to see Jesus through your kindness, and later we decided we wanted to be like Jesus too."

Jesus walked over and said, "All the times that you said you were not educated enough to teach a class, that all you could do was hand out snacks, you never knew you were actually handing out love. Some of these kids had no mother, or at least not a mother who truly loved them. To them, you represented the love that Jesus showed to people. You took seriously what I had taught: that to give things in My name was the same as giving them to Me. This is the result."

Next, a dirty, unshaven man slowly walked over. He said, "I no longer look like this. I wanted to let you see me the way you saw me on earth." It took a few seconds before Ollie remembered that the man had approached her for a handout once when she was on vacation. He filled in the story for her. He said, "I was an addict and alcoholic, and I was searching for someone to give me enough money to continue my high. At first you said you didn't think you had any money, and I thought you were just trying to get rid of me. Then I saw your eyes, and I felt as if you could feel my pain. You told about remembering nights you went to bed hungry as a child and young adult. You even apologized when all you could find was a dollar to give me. The compassion I saw in your eyes as you handed me the dollar along with the last words you said before you walked away haunted me. I could not get you telling me to use the money for food and not alcohol out of my head. The other words you said after that really touched my heart. You simply stated, 'God loves you, and if you trust Him, everything will be all right.' I tried several times to go into the liquor store, yet each time I approached the door, I heard your voice and saw your eyes and that sweet smile.

"I continued to walk around and saw a man offering rides to something called the rescue mission. I told them, 'Look, I have one dollar some lady gave me. She told me to use it for food, and she said something about God loved me and could help me. Can I give you this dollar to get me to this mission place to find some food?' The man responded, 'Better than that. You can get a real meal and keep your dollar.' That night I heard for the first time about God's love for the unlovable, even someone as unlovable as me. I remembered your words and sincerity and decided that if knowing this God produced someone like you, then I wanted to know Him also. I gave my heart to Him that very night and entered their program. I was able to get back on my feet, get clean, and return to work. I even went on to establish a ministry for the homeless living out on the street. The ministry I founded eventually led thousands to Christ, and many were no longer on the street as a result. It all started with your unselfish act and just a few kind words. You were the only person who didn't either judge me, push me away, or spit on me. You treated me like a human, something no one had done for a very long time. I just wanted to meet you and let you know you had made a difference."

 A few more people came over to share their stories, and all Ollie could do was just sit in amazement. She said, "I didn't do anything. I never stood in front of a congregation to preach, never taught a class, was not very good at witnessing. How can these people think I did anything?" Jesus smiled and said, "You see, it was Me who worked through you. I could not do that unless you were willing to allow Me to work. You made yourself available for service. You didn't think you had any talent or special gifts, yet you were willing to show others what I looked like by the way you lived your life. You were willing to do what you could with what you had. You gave everything to Me, and I in turn used that to reach so many. I, too, wish to thank you. "Now I want to take a break and let you see a few other people before you hear more of these stories." Suddenly she saw her parents, her in-laws, and her husband. They enjoyed a time of reunion and shared many stories and remembered many good times. After enjoying the time together, Bob said, "Someone has been waiting patiently to see you." A smiling, blue-eyed boy stepped up and yelled, "Momma!" as he threw his arms around her neck. Ollie was so overwhelmed to finally be reunited with her son Steve. They embraced for a very long time, and the others walked away to give the two time to catch up. Steve told her there was one person she had not yet met, and he wanted to escort her there.

 Jesus came over and led both to a glorious throne. He looked over His shoulder and said, "You see the angels around the throne? You were right; they are real."

Immediately she fell on her face before the Creator of the universe, God Himself. She was amazed as she began to praise Him in song. Instead of only making a joyful noise, she now had a beautiful voice.

As exciting as meeting all the others had been, nothing could compare to this moment. Ollie now understood that everything she had read and heard about God and heaven was true. She was now truly living in paradise. Nothing she had endured during life seemed to matter. She was now face-to-face with her God. She had worshipped before during her life; however, now the worship was all her heart desired. It had all been true, and now she was living in that reality. If there were any message, she could send back to her loved ones still alive on earth, she would say, "It's all true, and I look forward to you experiencing it with me. I love you."

ABOUT THE AUTHOR

~

  Pastor and Author Roger R. Sigmon is a licensed minster engaging in ministry through writing, speaking and community outreach development. He has been involved in ministry for over 33 years. His passions have focused on international missions and domestically in community outreach and redevelopment. During this time, he has served in many volunteer assignments, ministered in twelve countries, served as a youth leader and as a campus pastor.

  He has founded or co-founded several ministries, including Trek-X-Treme, Reset4Life, Real Life Knox, Ministry Happens and is currently in the process of planting a worship/outreach experience known simply as B-Church.

  Sigmon is available for speaking engagements, weddings, funerals, revivals, and retreats. He is a bi-vocational pastor and makes his home with his wife Carol and daughter Gracie in East Tennessee. For more information on him and the afore mentioned ministries please visit www.Rogersigmon.com

MORE BOOKS FROM THE AUTHOR

~

Roger R. Sigmon is the author of three previous books. These are all available through most online book retailers such as Amazon.com

Soul Garden: Growing a Stronger Relationship with God

ISBN-10: 1493517538

ISBN-13: 978-1493517534

Does God still work miracles? Do you have dreams and visions too far-fetched to even think about? God can make the impossible become possible. Soul Garden is a 16-week individual or small group study that will help develop spiritual disciplines which will enable you to focus more on God and others while making yourself more usable and available for what God has planned. Just as soil needs to be prepared before planting a garden, our hearts need to be prepared likewise to receive God and His word. If you are ready to get serious about making a difference in the world, then roll up your sleeves and begin preparing and growing your soul garden.

B-Church: Jesus Has Left the Building

ISBN-10: 150069911X

ISBN-13: 978-1500699116

Today's church seems to have lost focus on its mission of connecting people with Jesus. Instead of hiding behind the four walls of a building, Christ-followers need to be out engaging the community. Seeking out the broken, lost, and hurting and showing them Jesus in action. As Christ-followers we need to follow the example set by Jesus and meet people where they are. The only way to saturate society with the love of Christ is to actively engage those around us. We must go to them, not sit on a pew waiting for them to come to us. Don't just go to church Be the Church!

   Restore: The Jesus Flip

ISBN-13:978-1536877441

 Flipping houses has become a popular trend over the past several years. This is acquiring a run-down home and adding value through restoration or renovation, then selling for a profit. What would a life flipped by Jesus look like?

The steps to restoring a life or a home are very similar. This book shows the application of applying these steps to restoring a life. Jesus can take a life that seems wasted and worthless to others and transform it into something valuable and breathtaking. No life is beyond hope.

THANK YOU!!

www.ingramcontent.com/pod-product-compliance
Lightning Source LLC
Chambersburg PA
CBHW070800240726
48654CB00007B/148